HEALTH AMERICA

By Thomas J. McDevitt, M.D.

ISBN 0-933046-07-3

Little Red Hen, Inc.
P.O. Box 4260
Pocatello, Idaho 83205-4260

HEALTH AMERICA

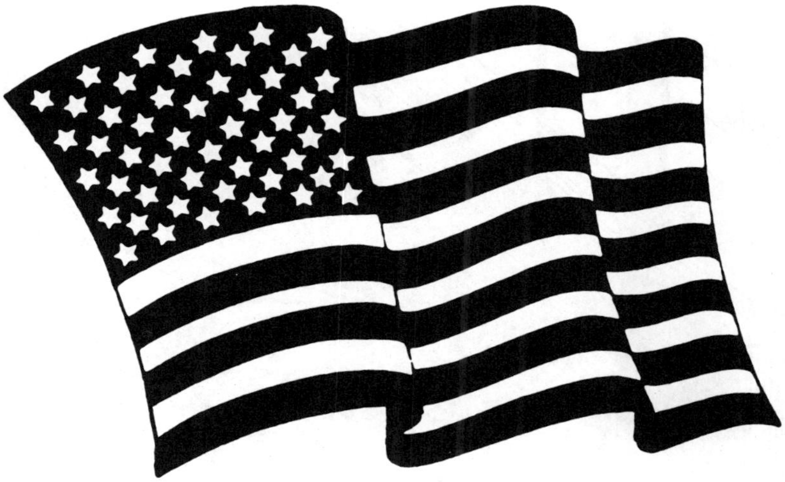

THE NERVOUS SYSTEM

Chapter 26

Thomas J. McDevitt, M.D.

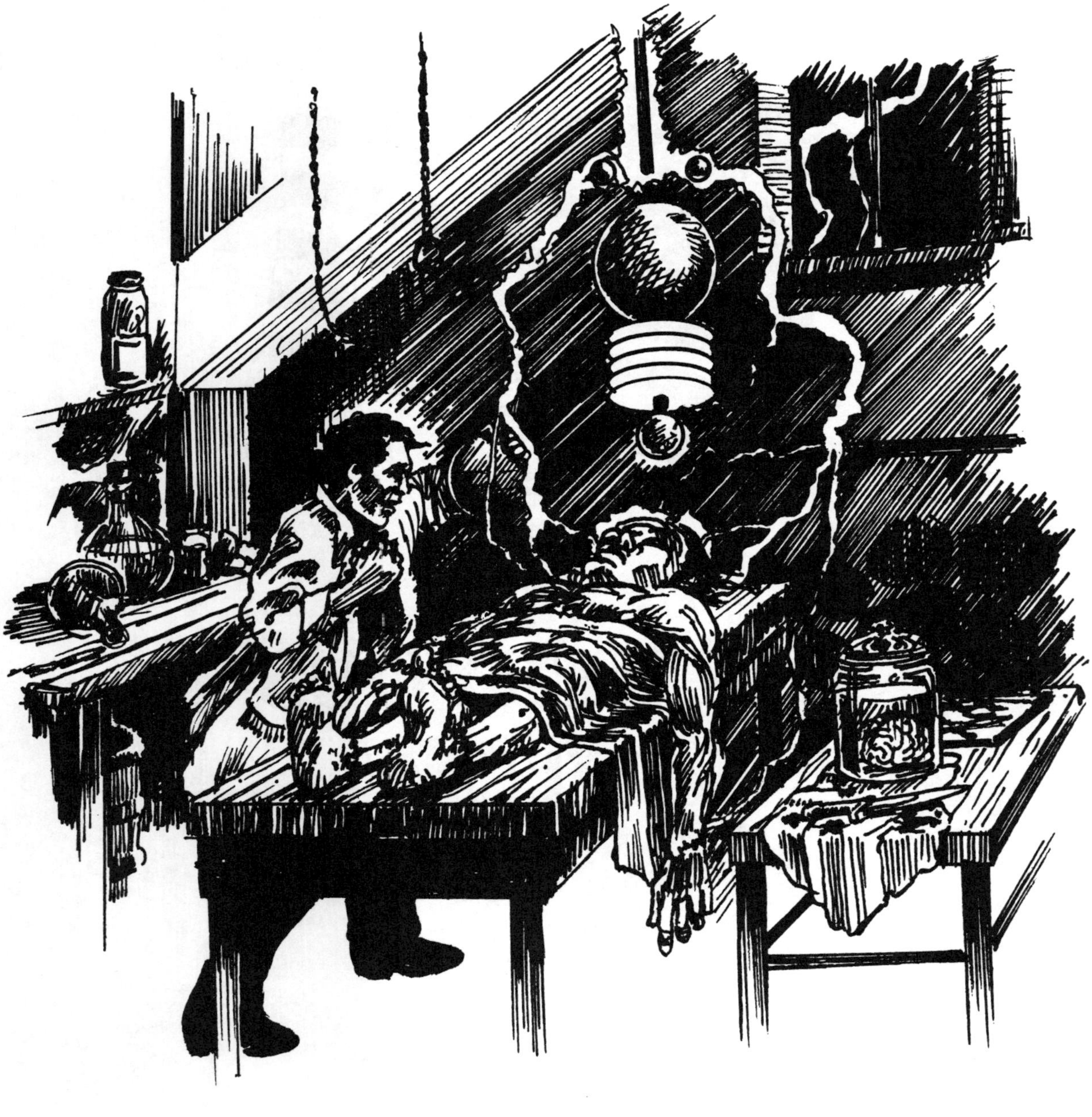

HEALTH AMERICA
CHAPTER 26

Table of Contents

CHAPTER 26

THE NERVOUS SYSTEM

"We may thank heaven that we have something better than our brains to depend on."
Lord Chesterfield

INTRODUCTION

Life begins as a single cell. This cell divides into two and these two into four. Finally, your body is made up of millions of cells. Some of these cells become nerve cells. Taken together the nerve cells comprise the nervous system.

CENTRAL, PERIPHERAL

Your nervous system has two major parts or "**systems**." Those nerves in the brain and spinal cord make up the **central** nervous system. Those nerves outside the brain and spinal cord make up the **peripheral** nervous system.

THEIR JOB

Because of nerves, your body parts work together. Your brain has your mouth stick out your tongue. It lets your thumb scratch your nose. In effect, the nervous system is like a giant telephone system that keeps the cells in touch with each other.

THE NEURON

BOTTOM LINE

In business, people ask, "What is the bottom line?" After all the facts and figures are seen, they want to know what it all means. In the nervous system, the bottom line is the **neuron.**

The neuron is the little gray cell where it all happens. It is the basic unit of the nervous system. The neuron relays nerve impulses, sending them in all directions. It decides which impulses may pass and which are blocked. Each of us may have one hundred billion neurons.

AFFERENT, EFFERENT AND INTERNEURONS

We have three types of neurons. **Afferent** or sensory neurons send messages **TO** the brain or spinal cord. **Efferent** or motor neurons take messages **AWAY** from the brain or spinal cord. **Interneurons** take messages from an afferent neuron to an efferent neuron. Interneurons are in the gray matter of the brain or spinal cord.

BODY, DENDRITE AND AXON

The three main parts of a neuron are: cell body, dendrite and axon. As arms and legs are to your body, so are the dendrites and axons to the neuron's cell body.

The **cell body** contains the nucleus. This is a small, round mass of tissue. Without a nucleus, the cell cannot grow. The nucleus also holds the traits we inherited from our parents.

Dendrite: Dendrite means tree. A neuron's dendrites are short stubby branches. A neuron sometimes has one, but usually several dendrites. The job of the dendrite is to receive signals and bring them into the cell. Among the many signals that a dendrite may receive are ones of sight, smell or touch.

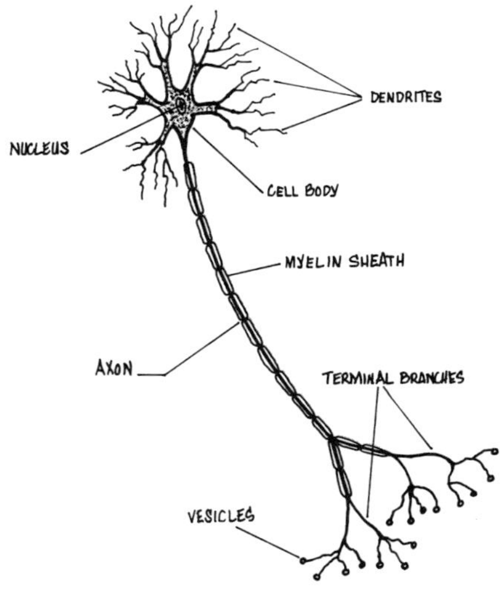

Fig. 1 Neuron

Axon: The third main part of a neuron is the axon. The axon carries signals away from the neuron's cell body. If the dendrites are the branches of the neuron, then the axon is its root. A neuron has only one axon. Groups of axons traveling together in a bundle form a **nerve.**

Outside the brain, most axons are covered with a coat called **myelin**. The myelin insulates the axon so that electricity flowing down the axon does not leak out the sides.

In a man's leg, axons may be three feet long. In a whale, they may be thirty feet long. Near their ending, axons split into little branches. The ends of these branches have bags called **vesicles**. Inside the bags are chemicals which leak out and send messages to the next nerve, muscle, or gland.

HOW NEURONS WORK

Specialists: Neurons are specialists. This means that each neuron has only one job. The job may be to hear a sound or make a muscle twitch.

An example might be if you stepped on a tack. A pain dendrite in your foot would take the message to the neuron cell body (afferent, sensory). Then the cell body would send a message down its axon to nerves in your spinal cord.

One spinal cord neuron (efferent, motor) would send a message down its axon to a leg muscle. Your foot would jerk away.

Another spinal cord neuron (afferent) would send a message up its axon to your brain telling it that your foot has been injured.

A brain neuron (efferent) would send a message to your throat muscles about the accident. You would say, "Ouch!"

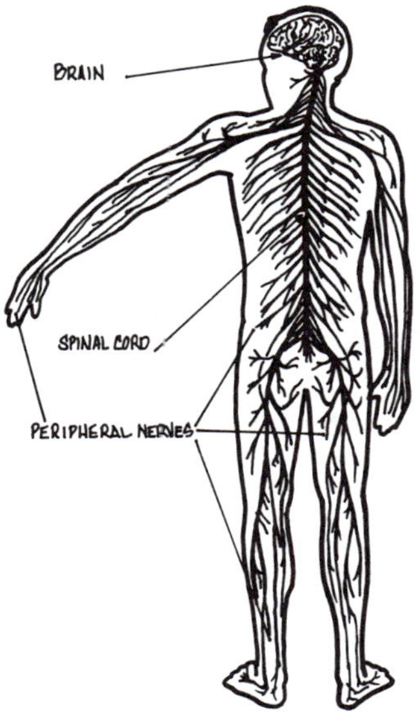

Fig. 2 Nervous System

ELECTRICITY AND CHEMICALS

To deliver a message, the neuron sends an electrical charge down its axon. When the axon approaches the next neuron, the electrical charge goes into all of its little branches. The electricity then causes the chemicals from the vesicles to seep out and enter the dendrites of the next neuron. The leaking of the chemicals and contact with the next nerve's dendrites is a **synapse.**

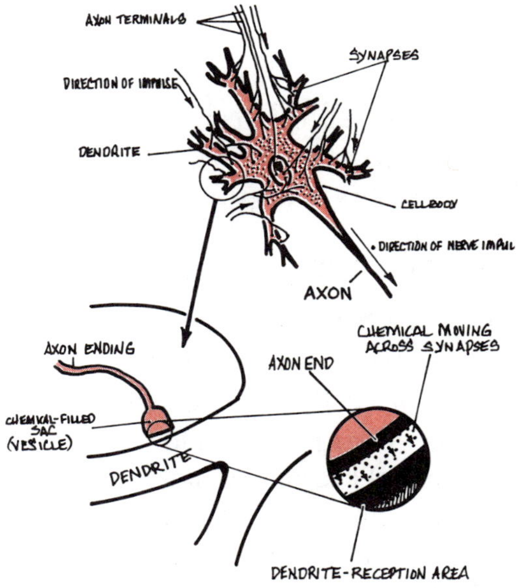

Fig. 3 Synapse

The chemicals in this synaptic process are **transmitters.** For a time, we thought that there were only one or two chemical transmitters. Now we know that there may be hundreds of different kinds. Two important chemical transmitters are acetylcholine and norepinephrine, also called noradrenaline.

Messages from neurons go only in one direction. They arrive at the dendrite, go through the cell body and down the axon. They cannot back up.

ALL OR NONE

A neuron must receive a strong enough message or stimulus for it to fire. This is the **"all or none"** law. If a single neuron receives a very weak message, it may not work.

A weak message may cause only a few neurons to fire. A strong stimulus would cause many neurons to fire. This explains the difference between a little hurt and a big pain, a fly on your nose and a lump on your head.

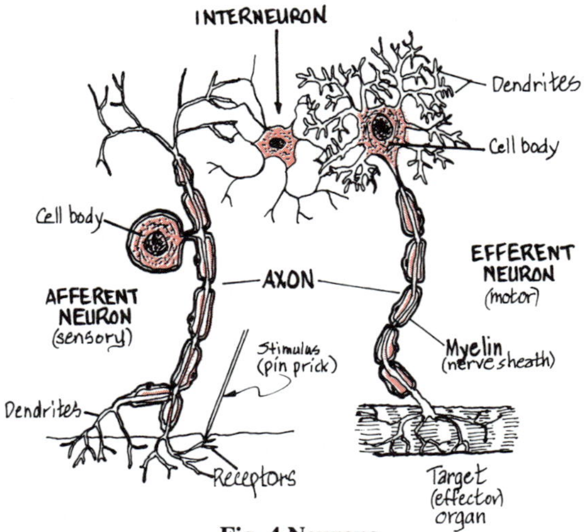

Fig. 4 Neurons

Although we have billions of neurons, they do not reproduce. You are born with all the neurons you will ever have. The neurons stop growing when you reach about the age of fifteen. If, from injury, age or drugs, a neuron is killed, it will never regrow.

NEUROGLIA

Besides neurons we have another type of cell in our nervous system. These are the **glial (neuroglia)** cells. There are nine times more neuroglia cells in your nervous system than there are stars in the sky. That is over 900 billion cells.

ASTROCYTES, MICROGLIA, OLIGODENDROGLIA, AND SCHWANN CELLS

There are four types of glial cells. The star-shaped **astrocytes**, (astros means star, and cyte means cell), are in the brain. These cells form tight bands around the brain's blood vessels. Their job is to allow water, oxygen, carbon dioxide and alcohol to reach the brain neurons but keep larger molecules out. This is the **"blood-brain barrier."** The blood-brain barrier is important when it comes to giving medicines to combat brain infections. The doctor must be sure the medicine he gives can pass through the blood-brain barrier.

Microglia are small cells that do not seem to do much until an infection occurs. Then they enlarge and move around and eat bacteria and dead matter.

Oligodendroglia are glue cells. They help the various nerve cells stick together. They also form the myelin sheath that surrounds nerve fibers.

Schwann cells are glial cells found only in body nerves. They are not in the brain or spinal cord. They help form two sheaths which cover nerves outside the brain and spinal cord.

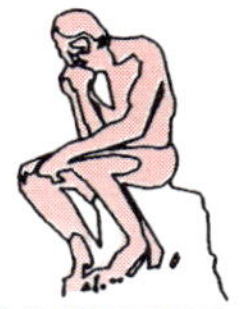

CONSIDER 26:1
MULTIPLE SCLEROSIS (MS)

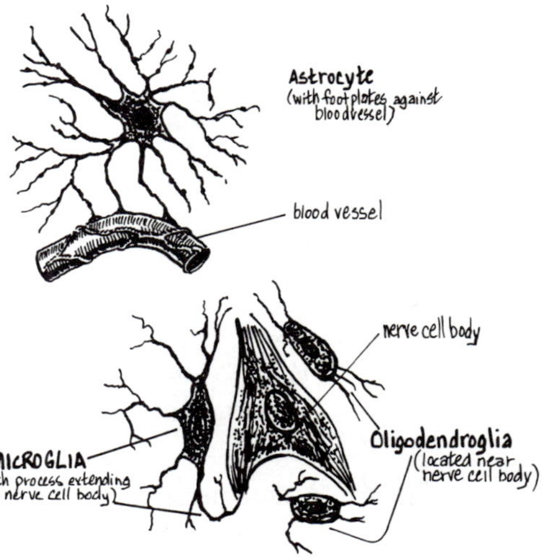

Fig. 5 Glial Cells

As you know, the oligodendroglia cells make up the myelin sheath that covers the nerves outside the brain. A disease of this glial cell is multiple sclerosis or MS. In this problem, the myelin sheath covering the nerve is destroyed. Because of this, electrical impulses can no longer travel down the nerve. Slowly the nerve dies. There may be loss of vision, dizziness, and slurred speech. A doctor named Charcot described three symptoms which happen with multiple sclerosis and are called Charcot's triad. The three symptoms are nystagmus (jerky eyes), tremor (shaky hands) and slurred speech.

Because the disease has a very slow onset and the symptoms may come and go, multiple sclerosis is a hard disease to diagnose. The first signs are usually a funny feeling in a hand or foot or one side of the face. There may be clumsiness of a leg or hand. The person may also have partial blindness and pain in one eye.

Those with multiple sclerosis usually spend the last years of their life in a wheel chair.

The cause of multiple sclerosis is not known and there is no cure. Multiple sclerosis may last twenty years or longer. It is most common in females 20 to 40 years of life.

****

SUMMARY
THE NEURON

The nervous system allows the body's cells to work together. The basic unit of the nervous system is the neuron. The neuron has a body, dendrites and a single axon.

There are three types of neurons. Afferent or sensory neurons send messages **to** the brain or spinal cord. Efferent or motor neurons take messages **from** the brain or spinal cord. Interneurons relay messages **from** afferent **to** efferent neurons. The neurons communicate with each other through a chemical mechanism known as a synapse.

In addition to neurons, the nervous system contains billions of neuroglial or glial cells. The duties of the four types of glial cells are to form the blood-brain barrier, hold the neuronal cells together, form the myelin and other nerve sheaths, and eat bacteria and dead tissue.

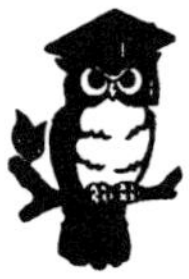

POP QUIZ:1
THE NEURON

Circle the correct answer

1. The brain, spinal cord and nerves comprise the:
   A. nervous system B. skeletal system C. astrocytes
   D. motor neurons

2. A neuron is made up of a cell body, dendrites and:
   A. astrocyte B. myelin sheath C. axon D. glial

3. There are three types of neurons: afferent, efferent and:
   A. motor B. sensory C. mixed D. interneuron

4. The chemical transfer between two neurons is called a:
   A. synapse B. acetylcholine C. norepinephrine
   D. transference

5. Neuroglia or glial cells may:
   A. form nerve sheaths B. form the blood-brain barrier
   C. hold neurons together D. all of the above

True or False

6. A bundle of axons is what we call a nerve:
   T. F.

7. Nerve impulses travel in only one direction:
   T. F.

8. The "all or none law" says that in order for a neuron to fire it must have a strong enough impulse:
   T. F.

9. Only a few nerves firing gives a mild sensation:
   T. F.

10. Pain going from your toe to your spinal cord travels by way of an efferent neuron:
T. F.

PERIPHERAL NERVOUS SYSTEM

AUTONOMIC NERVOUS SYSTEM

When we wink at a friend, it is a voluntary action. We make it happen. Also, to kick a ball is a voluntary action.

However, bodily functions must go on by themselves. It would be terrible to have to think every time you needed a breath, or to make your heart beat. These functions are **autonomic**. The part of our nervous system that controls these actions is the **autonomic nervous system.**

When your stomach rumbles, it is because of your autonomic nervous system. If you are frightened and your hair stands on end, it is because of the autonomic nervous system.

The autonomic nervous system is part of the general nervous system which we have been studying. It has parts which are within the brain and spinal cord, and so is part of the central nervous system. It has fibers outside the brain and spinal cord, so is part of the peripheral nervous system. The autonomic nervous system is usually considered a division of the **peripheral nervous system**.

All the fibers of the autonomic nervous system go from the central nervous system to the organs or muscles that they stimulate. Therefore, all the nerves of the autonomic nervous system are **efferent** or motor nerves.

The following structures are regulated by the autonomic nervous system:

Heart muscle
Blood vessels
Bronchial tubes
Stomach
Gallbladder
Intestines
Urinary bladder
Spleen
Eye (iris and ciliary muscles)
Hair follicles
Sweat glands
Lacrimal glands
Digestive glands (salivary, gastric, pancreas, liver)
Adrenal medulla

The autonomic nervous system has two subdivisions. They are the **sympathetic system** and the **parasympathetic system.** Almost all of the above organs receive both sympathetic and parasympathetic nerves. In general, sympathetic nerves **stimulate** or speed bodily functions; parasympathetic nerves **inhibit** or slow bodily functions.

When we are in trouble, the sympathetic system takes control. When we are relaxed, the parasympathetic system is in charge. But the autonomic nervous system never lets us get completely out of control or totally relaxed. In other words, there is always some of both the sympathetic and parasympathetic nervous systems at work in all the organs. This establishes "**homeostasis**," a state of equilibrium or balance.

Axons of the autonomic nervous system meet outside the brain and spinal cord with other neurons. These knots of cells are **ganglia**.

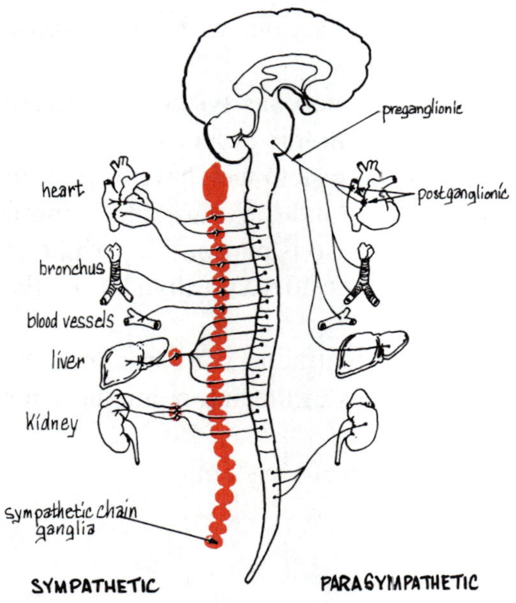

Fig. 6 Autonomic Nervous System

SYMPATHETIC SYSTEM

On each side of the front of the spinal cord from the second cervical (neck) vertebra down to the level of the tail bone (coccyx) are a series of ganglia. Short fibers connect the ganglia. Because they look like two chains of beads, they are often called the "**sympathetic chain ganglia**."

Before they meet with other neurons in the ganglia the nerve fibers are **preganglionic**. The dendrites and cell bodies of these neurons are in the chest (thoracic) and small of the back (lumbar) parts of the spinal cord.

The sympathetic ganglia then send out long (postganglionic) nerves. This is the **sympathetic** part of the autonomic nervous system. At the end of their axons, the fibers release the chemical norepinephrine or noradrenaline. Therefore, these nerves are **adrenergic**. The "ergic" part of the word means that they work with adrenalin.

The axons of any one preganglionic sympathetic neuron usually synapses with many postganglionic neurons which then go to many different organs. Therefore, the results of sympathetic stimulation are widespread: your hair stands on end, your mouth is dry, your heart races, etc. This is the **"fight-or-flight"** reaction and is similar to the rage reaction which we will study later.

PARASYMPATHETIC SYSTEM

The cell bodies of the preganglionic parasympathetic nerves are in the base of the brain and the lower part (sacral) of the spinal cord. Their axons are in cranial nerves 3, 7, 9, 10, 11 and some pelvic nerves.

These nerves from the base of the brain and lower back do not meet their ganglia until they are near the organ they stimulate. Often their ganglia are imbedded in the organ they wish to stimulate. So their preganglionic fibers are long and their postganglionic fibers are short. For example, the axons for fibers of the 10th (vagus) nerve arise in the base of the brain and travel over a foot before reaching their ganglia in the heart. Parasympathetic stimulation involves usually just one organ.

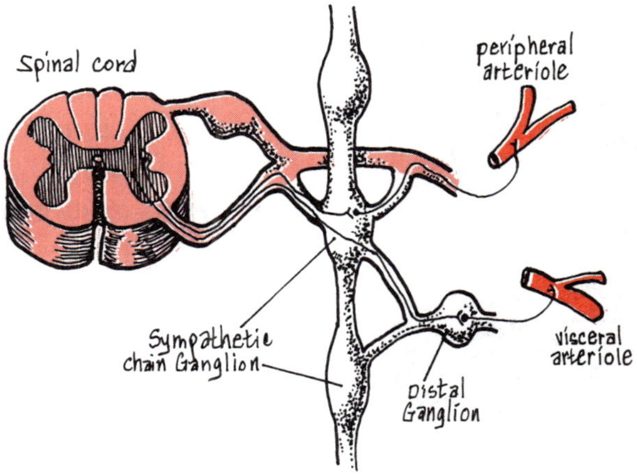

Fig. 7 Postganglionic Cell Body Endings In The End Organs And In The Sympathetic Chain Ganglia

These **parasympathetic** nerves release the chemical acetylcholine. They are cholinergic.

The autonomic nervous system does not always work by itself. If we wish, we can control our breathing. Some people can make their heart slow. Others decrease stress by telling their bodies to take it easy.

RAGE

An example of how the sympathetic nervous system works can be seen in the emotion, rage. In this emotion the sympathetic nervous system prepares the body for fight or flight as it sees fit. It is a period of intense **sympathetic** activity.

Things that may happen: extreme wakefulness, increase in muscular tone causing muscular tremor or spasms, elevated blood pressure, increased

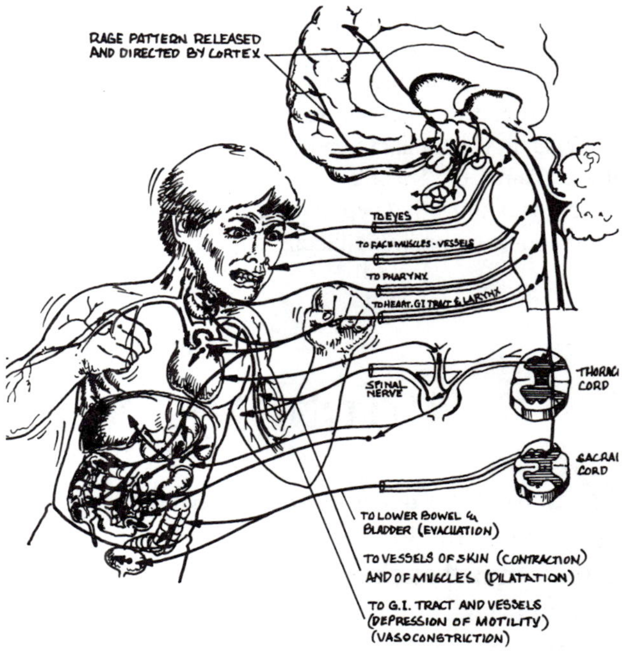

Fig. 8 Rage

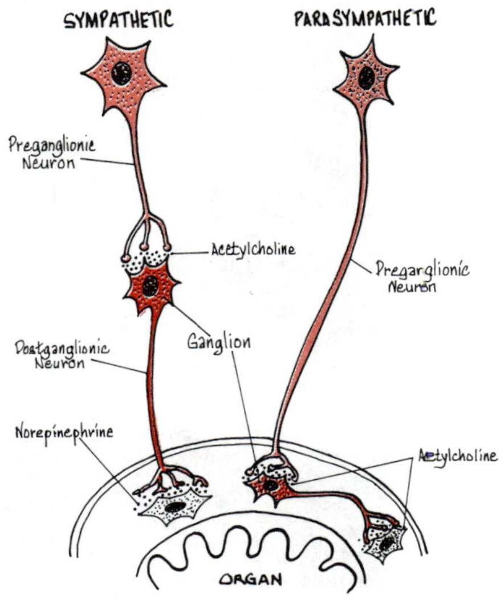

Fig. 9 Autonomic Nerve Innervations

blood volume, shift of blood from the stomach and skin to the muscles. The pupils of the eye become large then smaller. The nose runs. The throat becomes dry. The heart beats faster and stronger. The stomach feels tight.

Compare rage, a mostly sympathetic activity, to pleasure, a mostly **parasympathetic** reaction. In a state of pleasure the subject becomes sleepy. His gastrointestinal tract is normally and pleasantly active. He eats and rests with regularity.

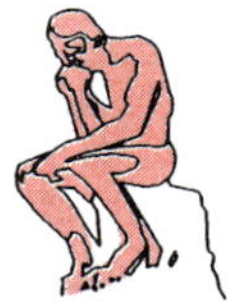

CONSIDER 26:2
STOMACH ULCER

Impulses to the stomach from the brain cause release of the chemical "pepsin" which aids in digestion. Normally, this occurs only during meals.

In people who develop stomach (peptic) ulcers, secretion continues between meals and at night. The tenth (vagus, wandering) nerve controls these secretions.

So the problem is due to abnormality of the parasympathetic system. These secretions eat away portions of the stomach, causing an ulcer crater and pain.

Emotions such as worry and anxiety increase the number of vagal impulses to the stomach. Peptic ulcer occurs commonly in persons who are under stress.

Because, in this case, the brain causes disease in a body part, peptic ulcer is a psychosomatic disorder.

What do you think of peptic ulcer? Do you know anyone who has such a problem? What part do you think "Tums" or "Rolaids" has in the control of this problem?

Did you know that peptic ulcer is now thought to be caused by bacteria and can be controlled by a short course of antibiotic therapy?

****

SUMMARY
AUTONOMIC NERVOUS SYSTEM

The autonomic nervous system controls those body functions which occur without our conscious knowledge. It is divided into two parts: sympathetic and parasympathetic. In general, sympathetic nerves **speed** body functions; parasympathetic nerves inhibit or **slow** body functions.

All nerves of the autonomic nervous system are motor efferent. The preganglionic cell bodies of the autonomic nervous system are in the gray matter of the brain or spinal cord.

Axons of the autonomic nervous system meet outside the brain and spinal cord with other neurons. These knots of cells are ganglia.

The ganglia of the sympathetic nervous system are in a series of connected ganglia alongside the spinal cord. These are the **sympathetic chain ganglia**. Ganglia of the parasympathetic nervous system are close to or imbedded in the organs which they stimulate.

The long postganglionic axons of the sympathetic nervous system release the chemical **norepinephrine** or noradrenaline. These nerves are adrenergic.

The parasympathetic nerves release the chemical **acetylcholine**. They are cholinergic.

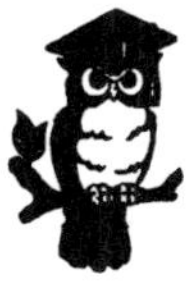

POP QUIZ:2

AUTONOMIC NERVOUS SYSTEM

Circle the correct answer

1. The part of the nervous system that handles unconscious impulses is called the ___________________ nervous system:
   A. sympathetic   B. parasympathetic
   C. autonomic   D. motor

2. One part of the unconscious nervous system is the:
   A. autonomic   B. motor   C. parasympathetic
   D. sensory

3. Another part of the unconscious nervous system is the:
   A. sympathetic   B. motor
   C. sensory   D. ganglionic

4. In general, sympathetic stimulation ___________ body function:
   A. slows   B. speeds   C. inhibits   D. stops

5. Parasympathetic axons secrete the chemical neurotransmitter:
   A. noradrenaline   B. norepinephrine   C. pepsin   D. acetylcholine

CENTRAL NERVOUS SYSTEM
BRAIN

We have likened your nervous system to a giant telephone company. By nerves, each of the millions of cells is linked together. This being so, then your brain is the central terminal, the main command box without which the system cannot work.

Your brain has the consistency of oatmeal mush. With your finger, you could poke a hole completely through your brain. Because of this, it must be protected against even mild injury. There are four protective mechanisms to protect the brain: scalp, skull, meninges and cerebrospinal fluid.

SCALP

Scalp means sheath. The scalp includes the skin, thick tissue under the skin, muscles going from back to front of the head, loose tissue under these muscles and a thick fibrous tissue over the skull.

The skin of the scalp is thicker than in any other part of the body. It has many blood vessels (vascular). If you cut your head, it bleeds a lot. Fortunately, by putting pressure on the wound, we can easily control the bleeding.

Connecting the muscle over the back of the head (occipital) with that over the front of the head (frontalis) is a thick band. This tendon is the **galea**. Galea means helmet.

SKULL

The skull has two parts, the **cranium** and the **face**. As we are now studying the brain, we will concern ourselves with the cranium. Cranium also means helmet.

Most of the 8 bones of the cranium are flat bones. The flat bones of the cranium give protection. They are two thin layers of compact tissue sandwiching between them a quantity of spongy tissue (cancellous).

In the cranium, these layers of bone are the **tables of the skull**. The outer table is thick and tough. The inner table is thinner, denser and more brittle (vitreous). The spongy bone between the two tables is the **diploe**. Diploe means fold.

Fractured skulls may be simple or depressed. Simple fractures on x-ray show a line across the bone where it was broken. A depressed fracture, such as if someone falls on the top of his head, shows that a portion of the bone is pushing down against the brain.

If someone has a simple skull fracture, he can often be watched for a while to see if there is further injury. With a depressed fracture, emergency treatment to save life is usually necessary.

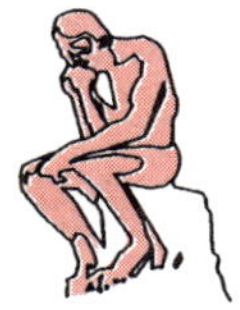

CONSIDER 26:3
BATTLE'S SIGN

Because the bone in the area is thick, a skull fracture at the bottom (base) of the skull is usually caused by a severe blow. These breaks do not often show up on routine skull x-rays or computerized scans.

However, bruising behind the ear (Battle's sign), black eyes (raccoon's eyes), drainage of clear fluid (cerebrospinal) from the nose, or blood behind the ear drum will suggest a broken head in this area. Not all these things need be present at the same time for there to be a fracture.

Skull fractures in this area may indicate severe underlying damage, consultation with a brain surgeon is indicated. Leakage of cerebrospinal fluid indicates a tear in the dura mater where bacteria may enter. Antibiotics may prevent infection.

****

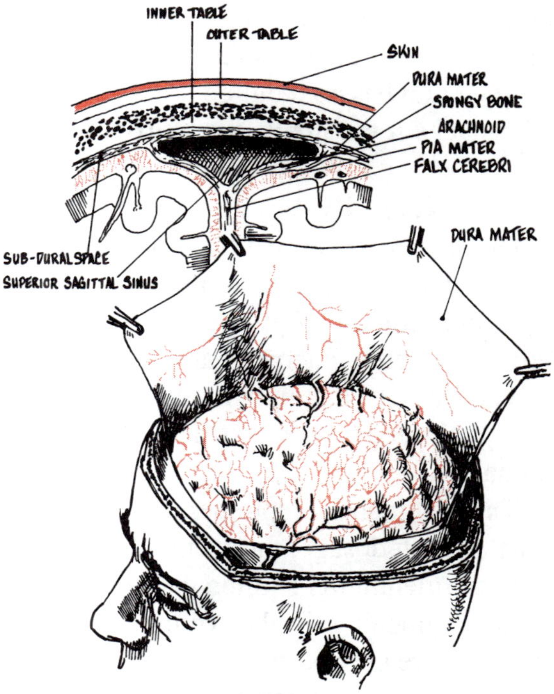

Fig. 10 Meninges

MENINGES

Meninges means membrane. There are three meninges or membranes which serve to protect the brain. These are an outer, tough fibrous membrane, the **dura mater**; a thin, middle, spider-web like layer, the **arachnoid**; and a soft, delicate inner covering, the **pia mater**.

DURA MATER: The outer cover is the dura mater. Dura mater means hard mother. The dura mater is thick and wants to cling to both the skull and the brain. The dura is also folded into four sickle-shaped folds, or processes called "falx", which go inward to the cavity of the skull to support and protect the brain. Between the folds of these septa are channels (**sinuses**) by which blood and excess cerebrospinal fluid are drained from the brain into the great veins of the neck. If there is blockage of this drainage, cerebrospinal fluid may build up in the brain, causing a condition known as hydrocephalus, or water on the brain. On the outer surface of the dura mater are arteries and veins that supply nutrition to the bone.

Infection and bleeding inside the skull may be outside the dura or inside the dura. If the bleeding is outside or between the dura and skull or backbone, it is called epidural. Epi means above. Bleeding here may put pressure on the brain and cause paralysis to the opposite side of the body.

If the bleeding is between the dura and brain or spinal cord, it is called subdural. Sub means below.

ARACHNOID: The middle brain cover is the arachnoid. Arachnoid means spider web. The arachnoid is so named because it is thin and transparent.

The dura mater adheres to the cranium. Its folds also go into the skull cavity. As we will see, the pia mater sticks to the brain. On the other hand, the arachnoid fits around the brain like a loose fluid-filled sack. The area between the arachnoid and the pia mater is the subarachnoid space. It is not really a space, as it is filled with spongy tissue and cerebrospinal fluid.

PIA MATER: Pia mater means tender mother. This is the cover that sticks closest to the brain. It follows the brain through all its folds. The pia mater is pierced by blood vessels going to the brain and spinal cord.

The brain has no feeling. It has no neurons that feel pain or temperature. When you have a headache it is usually due to irritation of the meninges or blood vessels.

MENINGITIS

Disease or inflammation of the meninges (dura, arachnoid, pia) is **meningitis**. Lepto means slender. Because of their thin and delicate nature, the arachnoid and pia mater taken together are the leptomeninges. Inflammation of the arachnoid and pia mater is leptomeningitis. Pachy means thick. Inflammation of the dura mater is pachymeningitis.

The cause of leptomeningitis is usually due to bacteria or viruses. Symptoms are: headache, pain in the back, stiffness of the neck and back, irritability and drowsiness ending in coma.

The treatment of leptomeningitis starts with a spinal tap to find the cause. Then, antibiotics in high dosage, intravenous fluids and oxygen are given.

Pachymeningitis is often the result of head wounds, sinus infection or ear infection. As with leptomeningitis, the symptoms are headache, pain in neck and back, stiffness and vomiting. There may be abscess formations and softening of the brain. X-rays are often necessary to discover the location of abscesses. Surgery may be indicated.

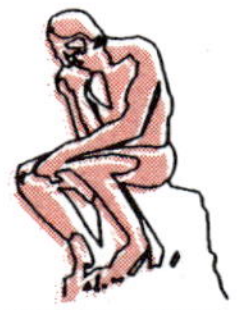

CONSIDER 26:4
THE YOUNG COP

A young cop in Atlanta, Georgia interviewed for a job. The chief said, "Here are four pictures. Look at the pictures. Tell me which of these people may pose the most trouble if arrested."

One picture was of a murderer. Another, of a bank robber. Then, there was a kidnapper, and last, a drunken old man.

The young cop studied the pictures, then handed them back to the chief. "I would be afraid to arrest the drunken old man," said the young cop.

The chief was surprised. The answer was correct. "Why did you choose the drunken old man?" He asked.

"Because," said the young cop, "alcoholics do not get enough vitamins. They bleed easily. They fall or hit their heads. Often, they bleed on the brain, then the blood clots. They have another accident and bleed again with more clotting. Over the years, these blood clots put pressure on the brain. A slight injury may be the last bleed that causes them to die."

What do you think of the young cop and his answer?

****

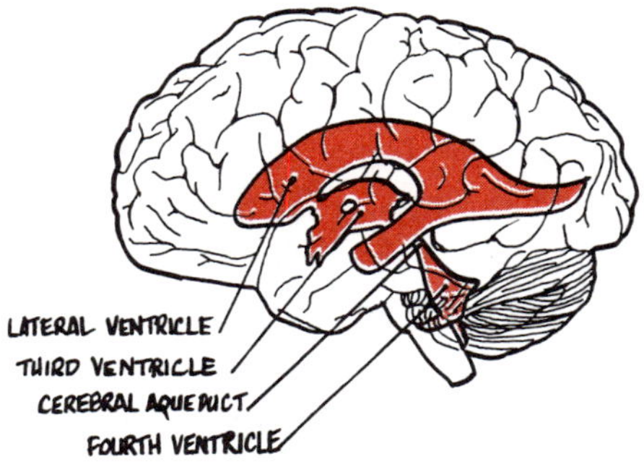

Fig. 11 Ventricles

CEREBROSPINAL FLUID

The cavity, which includes the brain and spinal cord, is a little less than two quarts. Of this volume, about one-quarter pint is cerebrospinal fluid. The cerebrospinal fluid is a watery cushion which protects the brain and spinal cord.

Cerebrospinal fluid is clear, colorless and odorless. Unlike blood, if left to stand, it does not clot. Usually the cerebrospinal fluid does not contain protein nor many cells. A bloody, yellowish, or cloudy color or the presence of protein in the cerebrospinal fluid suggests infection or injury to the brain or spinal cord.

The main purpose of the cerebrospinal fluid is to cushion the brain and spinal cord. Because the brain has about the same density as the cerebrospinal fluid, the brain is seen to float in this fluid. For this reason, a mild blow to the head will not usually damage the brain. A severe blow will not damage the brain on the side of the head on which it is struck. Instead, such a blow will cause the brain to rock to the other side where damage might occur.

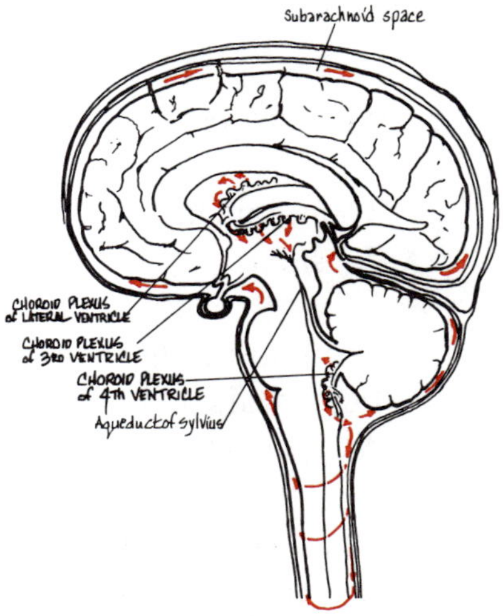

Fig. 12 Choroid Plexus

CIRCULATION

Inside the brain are four cavities called **ventricles**. Ventricle means little belly.

There are two lateral ventricles, a third ventricle and a fourth ventricle.

In each ventricle is a tuft of tissue called a **chorioid plexus**. Chorioid means skin-like and plexus means braid. It is in the chorioid plexus that spinal fluid forms.

Cerebrospinal fluid flows from the lateral ventricles into the third ventricle. It then goes through a tunnel (**aqueduct of Sylvius**) into the fourth ventricle. From the fourth ventricle, some fluid continues down the **central canal** in the spinal cord. The rest of the fluid slowly moves around the subarachnoid space of the brain and spinal cord.

SUMMARY
BRAIN PROTECTION

The brain is the central control unit for our nervous system. Because it is so fragile, it has four protective mechanisms: scalp, skull, meninges and cerebrospinal fluid.

The three meninges are the dura mater, arachnoid and pia mater. The dura mater adheres to the cranium and also sends folds into the skull called falx. Beneath the arachnoid, in the subarachnoid space, is a spongy tissue through which circulates the cerebrospinal fluid. The pia mater covers the brain and spinal cord closely through all their folds. Inflammation of the meninges causes the disease meningitis.

The cerebrospinal fluid's main function is to cushion the brain. It forms in the chorioid plexus of the four ventricles of the brain. Normally, the cerebrospinal fluid is clear, colorless and odorless.

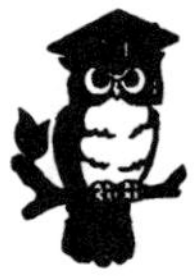

POP QUIZ:3
BRAIN PROTECTION

Circle the correct answer

1. Your brain has a consistency of:
   A. stone B. diamond C. mush D. bone

2. The four mechanisms to protect your brain are the meninges, cerebrospinal fluid, scalp and:
   A. circulation B. hair C. skull D. spinal cord

3. There are how many meninges:
   A. one B. two C. three D. four

4. The pia mater sticks closely to the:
   A. skull B. brain C. circulation D. chorioid plexus

5. The subarachnoid space is found between the:
   A. dura and arachnoid B. arachnoid and pia
   B. skull and dura C. pia and brain

THE BRAIN INTRODUCTION

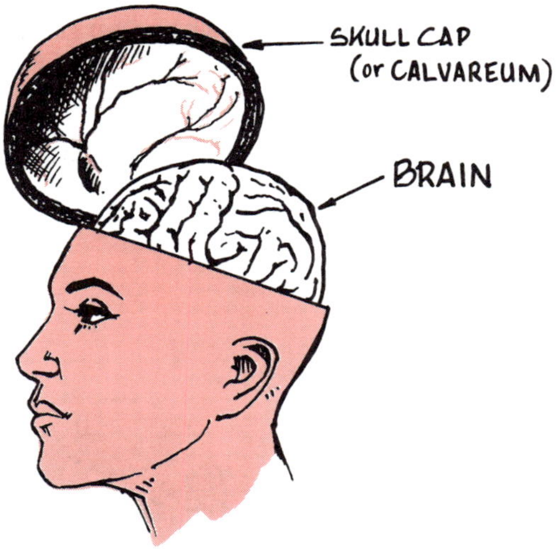

Fig. 13 The Brain

All animals have "brains", even a worm or snail. In lower animals it is just a thickened length of nerve. As animals get bigger and more complicated, so do their brains.

The human brain is the most complex tool in the world. No computer or animal brain can compare with the human brain in its ability to think, to reason, to learn and to remember. Language, thought, emotion and awareness of self are what make man different from animals and machines.

Your brain is the most important part of the central nervous system. It is the control center of your body. Almost all your activities and movements are controlled by your brain. It controls not only voluntary or conscious acts such as walking and talking but also skilled movements such as writing, typing and playing the piano. Even unconscious or involuntary acts such as coughing, blinking, swallowing, breathing and the heartbeat are regulated by the brain.

In addition to directing these activities, your brain is the seat of your emotions. If you are afraid, angry, jealous, or think you are in love, it is because of your brain.

Every thought, every feeling, every act, and every bodily function in our lives is ruled by the large mass of nerve cells that we call the brain. Your brain works all the time to keep you warm, upright and breathing.

EMBRYOLOGY

An embryo is the early growth stage of an individual. In the human, this stage is from the end of the first week of conception until the end of the second month.

Embryology is the science that deals with the growth of the embryo. A knowledge of embryology is important to the understanding of form and function of the human body. We will briefly study the embryology of our nervous system.

THE BEGINNING

We all start out as a single celled egg in our mother's womb. Immediately after fertilization by the male sperm, this egg begins to divide, first into two cells, then four, eight and so on to millions of cells. The process by which one cell divides into two or more is called **mitosis.**

Shortly after mitosis begins, three distinct cell layers are formed. These layers are the **entoderm**, **mesoderm** and **ectoderm**. These layers are spoken of as the **germ layers** of the embryo.

The entoderm will become your tonsils, stomach, liver, intestines, and lungs. The mesoderm will become your heart, blood vessels, skeleton, and muscles. The ectoderm will become your hair and nervous system.

NEURAL PLATE

During the early formation of the germ layers, there appears a thickening of part of the ectoderm. This is the neural plate.

The sides of this neural plate grow up and around the mid portion, forming what looks like a straw. This is the **neural tube**. The inside of the neural tube becomes the ventricles of the brain.

The front of the neural tube enlarges and then bends on itself, becoming the brain. From the inside of some neural tube cells, processes grow out to become the nerves.

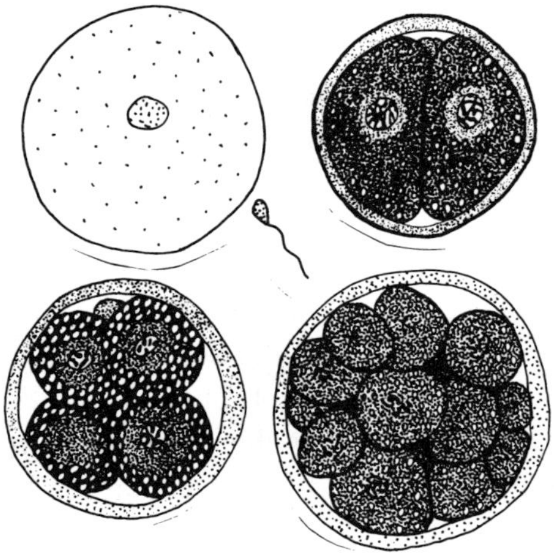

Fig. 14 Fertilization And Mitosis

PARTS OF THE BRAIN

The brain has three parts, the **forebrain**, prosencephalon; the **midbrain**, mesencephalon; and the **hindbrain**, rhombencephalon. The prefixes describe either the position (pros, meaning "before" or "in front of" and meso, meaning "middle") or shape (rhomb, from "rhombus," a mathematical figure).

The forebrain is further divided into the **cerebrum** and the **diencephalon**. The midbrain sits alone but is closely connected both above with the forebrain and below with the hindbrain. The hindbrain is divided into the **cerebellum** and the **brain stem**; the brain stem is composed of the **pons**, **medulla oblongata** and the **reticular activating system**. Each section of the brain is thought to have certain functions.

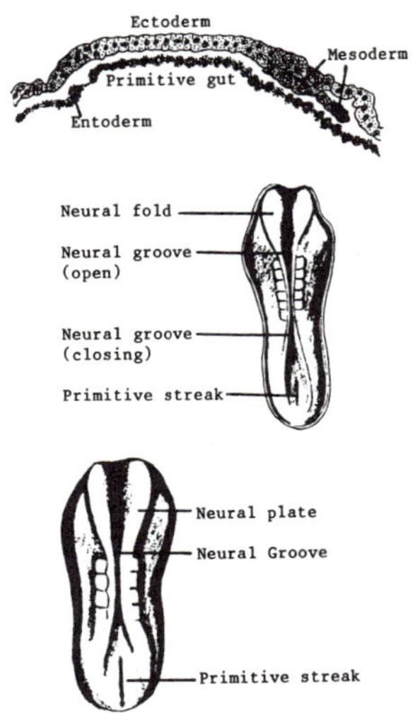

Fig.15 Division Of Germ Layers And Neural Plate

FOREBRAIN

* **Cerebrum**
  Cortex
  Basal Ganglia

* **Diencephalon**
  Thalamus
  Hypothalamus
  Pituitary Gland
  Limbic System

MIDBRAIN

HINDBRAIN

BRAIN STEM

* Pons
* Medulla Oblongata
* Reticular Activating System
  Cerebellum

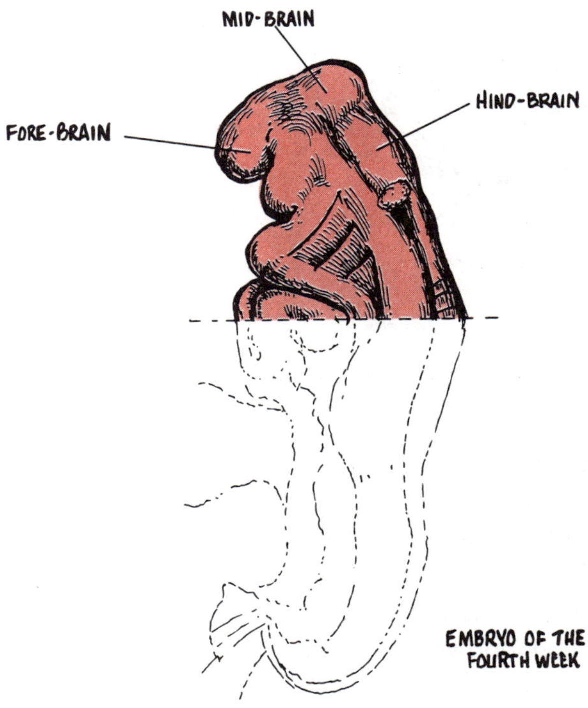

Fig. 16 Pig Embryo Of The Fourth Week

FOREBRAIN (PROSENCEPHALON)

CEREBRUM

Imagine that you could remove your brain and hold it in your hands. If you are a fifteen-year old girl, your brain is full size. You note that it weighs about three pounds. Tall persons have heavier brains than short persons. But, if you take the difference of size into account, short people have bigger brains than big people.

Your brain is soft. It feels like jelly or mush. It is gray in color.

GRAY MATTER: The reason that the brain looks gray is because that is the color of the billions of neurons and glia. This is the **gray matter**.

As we have studied, glia is a glue like substance that helps hold the brain together. In the brain, there are ten times more glial cells than neurons.

WHITE MATTER: Under the gray matter is the white matter. The **white matter** is made up of nerve fibers connecting different parts of the brain.

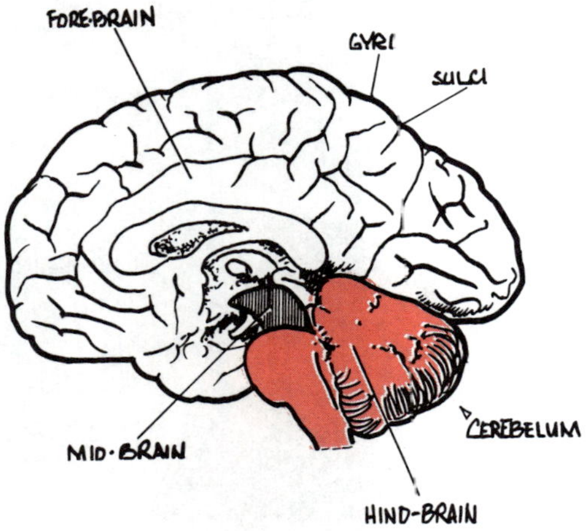

Fig. 17 Brain From The Side Cut In Two

CEREBRAL CORTEX: Cerebrum means brain. The outer layer of the cerebrum is the **cortex**. Down the middle and going from front to back is a deep groove. This groove is the **Great Longitudinal Fissure**. The great longitudinal fissure divides the cerebral cortex into two halves. These are the **hemispheres**. Hemi means half and sphere means ball.

CORPUS CALLOSUM: Deep to the great longitudinal fissure, the two cerebral hemispheres are connected by a mass of white matter. This is the **CORPUS CALLOSUM**. Corpus callosum means hard body.

The corpus callosum is white matter. It is made of nerve fibers. The job of the corpus callosum is to connect the hemispheres. If the fibers of the corpus callosum were cut, then one side of the brain wouldn't know what the other side was doing.

The cerebral cortex is wrinkled and looks like a walnut. The little wrinkles or grooves are **sulci**. The big wrinkles are **fissures**. The elevations between the sulci are **gyri**.

If you took your wrinkled cerebrum and spread it out, it would be the size of a card table. The wrinkles make you smart. The more wrinkles, the smarter you are. The reason for this is that the wrinkles let you have more room for gray matter.

Frogs, fish and snails have no wrinkles on their brains. Babies have some wrinkles. Teenagers have lots of wrinkles. When some people grow older, their wrinkles flatten out.

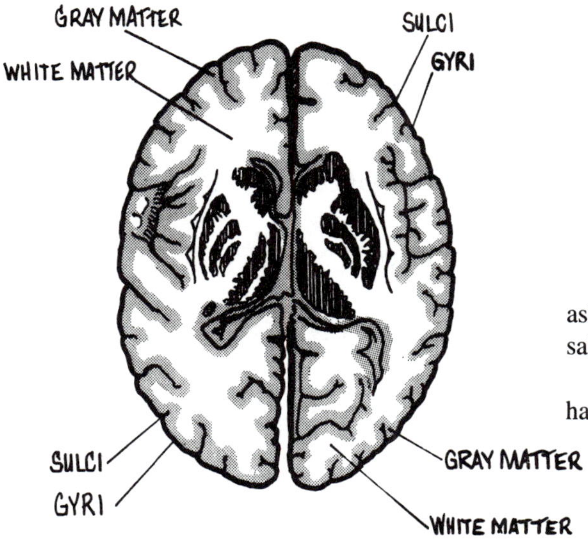

Fig. 18 Brain, Top View Cut In Half

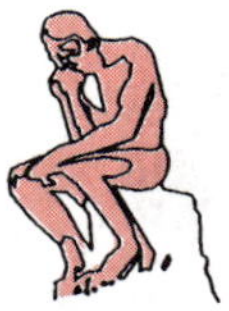

CONSIDER 26:5
NO GRAY MATTER

A girl in Austin, Texas did poorly on a test. When asked why she did so poorly, she tapped her head and said, "Not much gray matter."

What did the girl mean? Could she just as well have said, "Not many wrinkles."

****

SUMMARY
BRAIN, INTRODUCTION

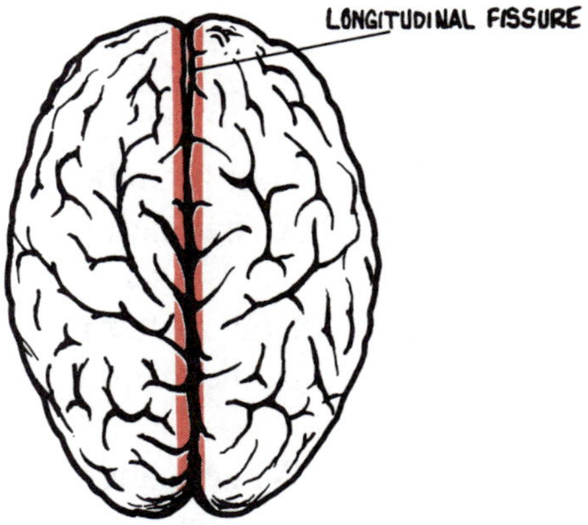

Fig. 19 Brain, Top View

Your brain is the most advanced communication system in the world. It controls conscious activities such as talking, as well as autonomic activities such as your heart beat.

The brain begins as a thickened layer of ectoderm called the neural plate. It forms a tube which then bends upon itself and enlarges. Processes grow out from the ectodermal cells to become nerves.

The brain has three parts: forebrain, midbrain and hindbrain. It is made up of gray matter and white matter. The gray matter is neurons and glial cells. The white matter is the axons of nerve fibers.

The largest part of the forebrain is the cerebrum. The outer layer of the cerebrum is the cortex. The cortex is wrinkled. The elevations of these wrinkles are gyri. The grooves are sulci. The deep groove dividing the cerebral cortex into two halves is the great longitudinal fissure. Each half of the cerebral cortex is a hemisphere.

Deep in the cerebral cortex is the corpus callosum. The corpus callosum is white matter which connects the two halves of the cerebral hemispheres.

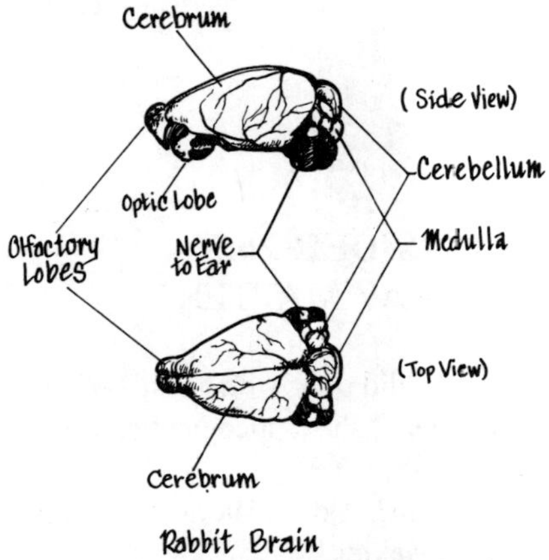

Fig. 20 Note Lack Of Wrinkles, Gyri And Sulci

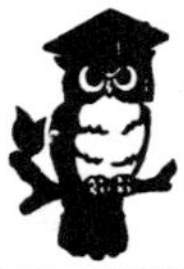

POP QUIZ:4

BRAIN, INTRODUCTION

Circle the correct answer

1. Your brain can be divided into how many parts:
   A. one B. two C. three D. four

2. The largest part of your brain is the:
   A. cerebrum B. midbrain C. hindbrain D. stem

3. The outer layer of the cerebrum is the:
   A. cortex B. white matter C. corpus callosum D. fissure

4. The raised folds on the brain are:
   A. gyri B. sulci C. fissures D. pons

5. Your brain begins as the:
   A. entoderm B. mesoderm C. glia D. neural plate

6. Gray matter is glial cells and:
   A. neurons B. entoderm C. mesoderm D. axons

7. White matter is:
   A. glia B. entoderm C. nerve fibers D. glia

LOBES

Each hemisphere of the cerebral cortex is made up of four lobes: **frontal**, **parietal**, **temporal** and **occipital**. Though connected, each lobe has its own job. Deep within the cerebral cortex is another mass of gray matter that some consider another lobe of the brain. This is the insula, central lobe or **Isle of Reil**.

FRONTAL LOBE: Behind the forehead are the frontal lobes. You think your greatest thoughts in the frontal lobes. Lower animals have either small frontal lobes or none at all.

The frontal lobes have much to do with **personality**. An injury, growth or infection in a frontal lobe may change a person's personality. Sometimes the change is for good, sometimes for bad. It is hard to say which way the change will go.

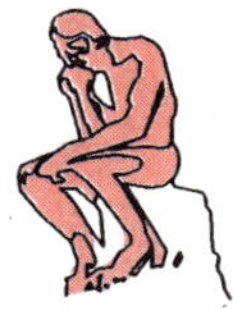

CONSIDER 26:6
TREPHINE

To trephine is to make a hole in the skull. This may be lifesaving. If someone falls and has bleeding inside his skull, it is important to make a trephine and let the blood out. This will relieve pressure on the brain.

In ancient times, Europeans and Indians of Peru thought that evil spirits in the skull caused mental illness. To release these spirits, the skull was trephined.

A round rock was used. The patient sat. The medicine man ground the rock into the sufferer's skull until a hole was made. There was little pain. Skulls in burial mounds show well healed trephine holes.

****

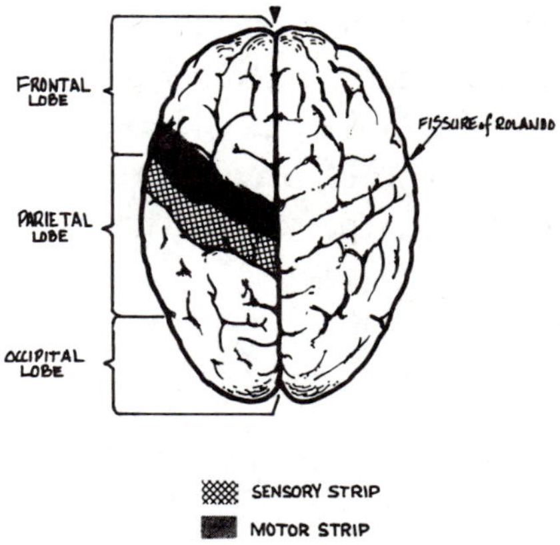

Fig. 21 Lobes, Top View

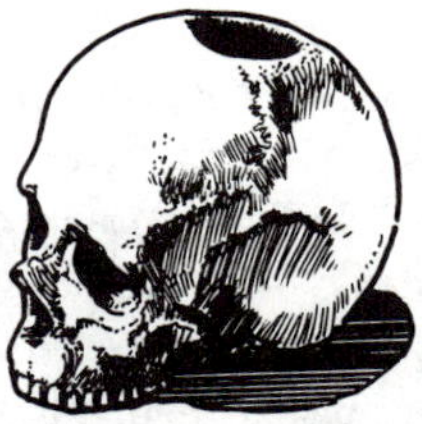

Fig.22 Ancient Trephine

MOTOR STRIP: At the back part of the frontal lobe is the **motor strip**. The motor strip has to do with **movement**.

If one part of your motor strip is touched with an electrical current, you may suddenly raise your arm. Another spot touched may cause you to cry out.

The size of the area on the motor strip concerning a certain function is related to how complex that part of the body is. Thus, the area for the face is bigger than the area for the leg. The area for the tongue is bigger than the area for the foot.

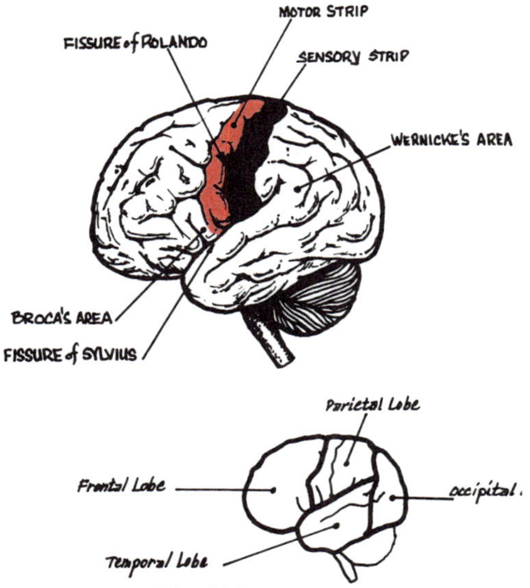

Fig. 23 Brain, Side View

An important area of the frontal lobe is **Broca's area**. It is found in the left hemisphere in almost all right-handed and most left-handed people. It is just in front of the lips-teeth-tongue area of the motor strip.

Broca's area **controls speech**. The area gets the information about what is to be spoken and plans the movements needed for speech production. It also arranges the motions needed for writing.

Broca's area has thousands of different laryngeal movements that are the patterns either of syllables or of whole words. It also probably performs the remaining tasks for producing the word. It controls the muscles of speech through the motor area of the larynx, jaw, and tongue and controls the muscles of respiration through closely allied areas on the surfaces of the frontal lobes.

A lesion of Broca's area causes trouble speaking and, in some cases, writing (motor aphasia). A person with this problem can say only very simple words such as "yes" or "no."

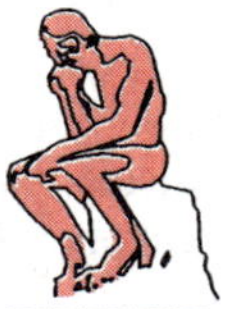

CONSIDER 26:7
PHINEAS GAGE

In 1848, at a stone quarry in Vermont, Phineas Gage was using a large medal rod to tamp blasting powder into a hole.

Suddenly a spark set off the powder. The four foot long rod shot up Phineas' cheek, through his brain and stuck out the top of his head. He was knocked out. A fellow worker was able to pull the rod out of Phineas' skull. The revived Phineas walked away.

Phineas suffered extensive injury to both frontal lobes of his brain. He could go back to work in the quarry, remembered everything, and was as good a worker as before.

There was a change however. Before, Phineas had been a foreman: pleasant, cheerful and liked by all. However, the new Phineas was different. He was irritable and fought with his fellow employees. He could no longer hold the job of foreman.

What do you think of Phineas Gage? What do you think of his injury? What does this tell you about the frontal lobes of the brain?

****

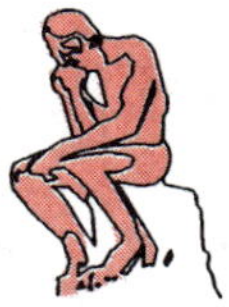

CONSIDER 26:8
PSYCHOSURGERY

In 1935 two doctors did an experiment on Chimpanzees. A chimpanzee named Becky would throw a temper tantrum whenever she made a mistake. The doctors made a small hole in Becky's skull. With a blunt knife they cut the connections between Becky's frontal lobes and the rest of her brain.

The results were startling. After the surgery, Becky made as many mistakes as before. Now, however, she no longer cared. It was as if she were in a happiness cult.

Lucy was another chimpanzee. Lucy was normal. She made mistakes but was always calm. Lucy had the same operation as Becky.

After her surgery, Lucy made many more mistakes. With each mistake, Lucy was upset. She screamed, banged on her cage, and stomped her feet.

What do you think of this experiment? Do you know that once this experiment was the basis of surgery on mentally ill people?

****

HOMEWORK 26:1
PSYCHOSURGERY

One Flew Over The Cuckoos' Nest is a book. It was later a movie. Go to the library and get this book or watch the movie.

What does this book have to do with what we are studying?

Write a report of at least three paragraphs about this book. Hand it in at the next class. Discuss your findings.

****

PARIETAL LOBE: At about the position of the front of your ears and going across the top of the brain from ear to ear is the **Fissure of Rolando**. This cleft separates the frontal from the **parietal lobes** of the brain. To the back are the parietal lobes. Parietal means the walls of a cavity. This refers to the inner, fluid-filled hollows of the brain called the ventricles which we have studied. The parietal lobes form walls for the main part of the ventricles.

At the front part of the parietal lobes, just back of the Fissure of Rolando, is the **Sensory Strip**. The sensory strip receives **feelings** such as touch, pain, temperature, taste, smell and size of objects.

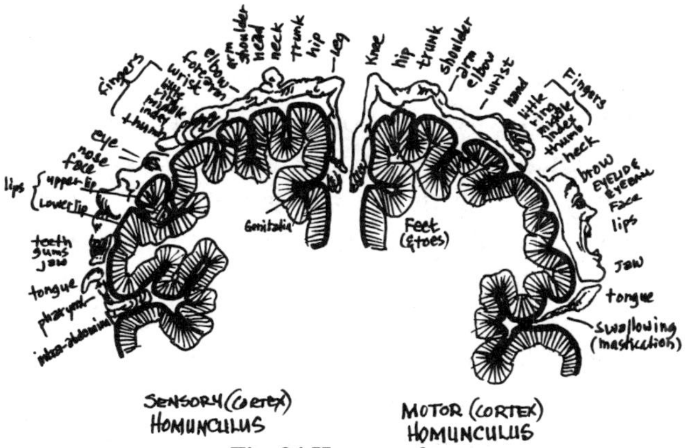

Fig. 24 Homunculus

From the sensory strip these feelings go to the **Angular Gyrus**.

The angular gyrus is in the lower part of the parietal lobe. It is in the angular gyrus that the brain puts together all the sensations coming to it from different parts of the body. In the angular gyrus thoughts about what is happening are formed.

For example, you eat a bowl of ice cream. You taste it. You smell it. You see it and feel the spoon going to your lips. These feelings all go to different parts of your sensory strip.

From the sensory strip they go to the angular gyrus. At the angular gyrus everything is put together: the taste, smell, sight and other feelings along with memory of what has happened before. Suddenly your brain says, "Hey, this is all right." The angular gyrus then sends a message to your motor strip and you lick your lips.

The angular gyrus is the place where you are able to interpret all the sensations coming to you at the same time. If an injury occurs to your angular gyrus, you may not understand the meaning of words that you hear or read. You may not be able to tell if an ice cube is hot or cold.

OCCIPITAL LOBE: In the back of the head is the **occipital lobe** of the brain. Occiput means just that, the back of the head.

The occipital lobes have to do with **vision**. Severe damage to this area may cause blindness. If you hit your head and cause slight damage to the occipital area, you may see stars.

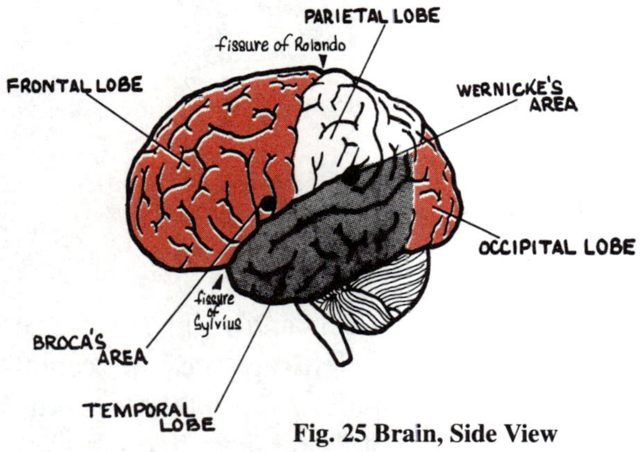

Fig. 25 Brain, Side View

TEMPORAL LOBE: On each side of the brain about the level of the ears and going from below to up and back is the **Fissure of Sylvius**. This cleft causes a part of the brain to look like the flaps on a hunting cap. These flaps are the **Temporal Lobes** of the brain. The temporal lobes have to do with **hearing**.

Wernicke's area is a large region of the parietal and temporal lobes of the left cerebral hemisphere. Among others, it contains parts of the angular gyrus.

Wernicke's area is thought to be essential for **understanding** and **making** sensible **speech**. It controls the ability to understand and use symbolism.

Wernicke's area is usually well developed in only one (the dominant) hemisphere. If you decide to speak, Wernicke's area forms your thoughts. The meaning of the word becomes understood here. Your choice of words begins in this area.

If you suffer damage to Wernicke's area of the cortex, you not only can't speak, but also can't read and understand spoken language. You may talk all the time, talking in gibberish with occasional mispronounced words. You may have difficulty naming objects, writing, reading, and calculating. You may not know which is the right or left. You may not seem to care about your condition.

INSULA: The insula or Island of Reil is deep within the cerebral cortex. It is sometimes called the **central lobe**. The insula can only be seen if the lips of the Sylvian fissure are widely separated. When a person has a stroke, the insula may cause **heart changes**. Damage to this area may also determine how soon a sufferer's hand may recover from the effects of a stroke.

SUMMARY LOBES

Each half of the cerebral cortex is made up of four visible lobes, plus one invisible mass of gray matter sometimes called the central lobe, insula or Isle of Reil. The four visible lobes are the frontal, parietal, occipital and temporal.

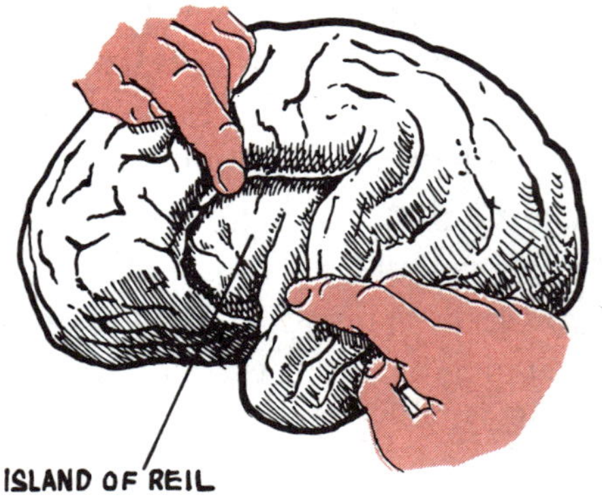

Fig. 26 Isle Of Reil

The frontal lobes have to do with your personality. Damage to a frontal lobe or its connections with other portions of the brain may profoundly affect a person's personality, sometimes for good, sometimes for bad. At the back of the frontal lobe is the motor strip. This area has to do with movement. Just in front of the motor strip is Broca's area, which deals with speech.

The parietal lobes are found at the top of the head behind the fissure of Rolando. At the front part of the parietal lobes is the sensory strip. The sensory strip receives feelings such as pain, taste, and heat. The sensory strip then sends these sensations to the Angular gyrus, which monitors them and then sends its results to other parts of the brain.

At the back of your head is the occipital lobe. The occipital lobe has to do with sight. Damage to the occipital lobe may cause blindness.

The temporal lobe is at the side of your head. It deals with hearing. Wernicke's area of the temporal and parietal lobes has to do with understanding and making sensible speech.

The Isle of Reil may deal with the heart effects of stroke and how soon a limb may recover from the effects of a stroke.

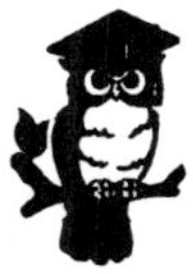

POP QUIZ:5
LOBES

Circle the correct answer

1. There are how many visible lobes of the brain:
   A. one B. two C. three D. four

True or False

2. The frontal lobe deals mostly with hearing:
   T. F.

3. Broca's area is found in the frontal lobe:
   T. F.

4. The sensory strip is found in the parietal lobe:
   T. F.

5. The parietal lobe deals mainly with sight:
   T. F.

6. The occipital lobe deals mainly with sight:
   T. F.

7. The fissure of Rolando separates the parietal from the occipital lobe:
   T. F.

8. The Sylvian fissure separates the frontal from the temporal lobe:
   T. F.

9. An intact Wernicke's area is necessary for understanding and making sensible speech:
   T. F.

10. The insula, central lobe or Island of Reil is thought to be important in determining how soon a person's hand might recover from a stroke:
    T. F.

BASAL GANGLIA

We know that ganglia means "knot." In the past, all knots or clusters of neurons or gray matter were known as ganglia. Then, after a while, those clusters of neurons or gray matter in the brain came to be called nuclei. Nucleus means nut or kernel. Ganglia refers to those clusters of nuclei outside the spinal cord and brain such as the sympathetic ganglia which we have studied.

Some clusters of gray matter in the brain have kept the name ganglia. In each cerebral hemisphere are several large knots of gray matter, called the **basal ganglia**. Sometimes they are called the basal nuclei. The basal ganglia include the **corpus striatum** (furrow), the **amygdaloid body** (almond shaped) and the **claustrum** (barrier). Other subdivisions of the basal ganglia are the **Putamen** (shell), **Caudate Nucleus** (having a tail), and **Lentiform Nucleus** (lens shaped).

<u>BASAL GANGLIA</u>

* Corpus Striatum
* Amygdaloid Body
* Claustrum

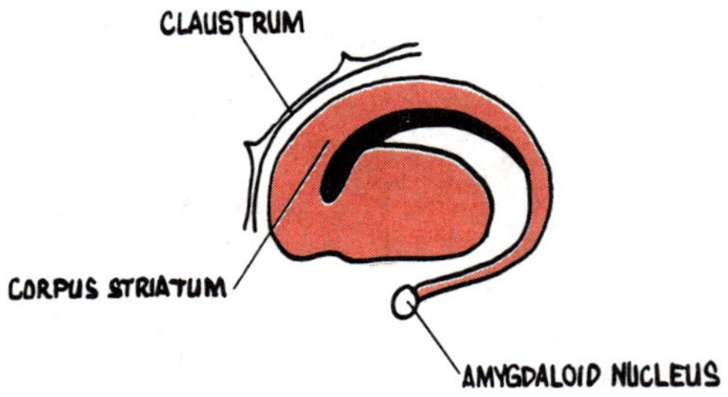

Fig. 27 Basal Ganglia

As with other portions of the nervous system, the basal ganglia start as small outgrowths of the primitive plate. However, the cerebral cortex grows and then folds back over other portions of the brain. The basal ganglia stay in approximately the same place. The result is that the ganglia come to lie below the cortex, deep within the white matter.

The basal ganglia are in charge of **complex patterns** and series of movements, especially slow, steady movements such as walking. It is also thought that the basal ganglia control activities that were once learned but are now done by **habit**. Examples of such activities include tying your shoes and eating.

The ganglia are interconnected by nerve fiber pathways. Nerve cells from all areas of the cerebral cortex send fibers to the basal ganglia. The basal ganglia send messages back to the cortex by way of the thalamus to control motor functions of the cortex. The normal operation of all these connections is vital for the smooth control of voluntary movements.

The basal ganglia are involved almost completely with **curbing actions** rather than with starting actions. This applies to all of the basal ganglia rather than to just some of them.

When the basal ganglia are stimulated by electrodes, very little or nothing happens. But when muscles are already in action, then stimulation of parts of the basal ganglia will stop the activity.

DISEASE OF THE BASAL GANGLIA

Tumors, viral and bacterial infections, blood vessel accidents, heredity and changes due to aging may cause disease in the basal ganglia. Some problems related to the basal ganglia are the following.

Athetosis:

Athetosis is a problem in which continual writhing movements occur in different parts of the body. This occurs especially in the hands and limbs as long as the patient is awake. For instance a person may show continual rhythmic contortions of a hand, an arm, or a shoulder. Sometimes the writhing movements involve one entire side of the body or both sides of the body.

Choreiform Movements:

Some children who have rheumatic fever develop sudden, jerky, uncontrollable movements. This problem is called St. Vitus' dance. More technically, it is Sydenham's chorea.

While the child is engaged in normal activity, different portions of his body will suddenly jerk to a new position. His head will suddenly turn, his eyes will suddenly jerk upward or downward. The movements continue as long as the child is awake. Fortunately, this usually goes away as the disease gets better.

In Huntington's chorea, a hereditary problem, nerve cells die. There is uncontrollable jerking movements, depression, irritability, and mental decay. The problem attacks both sexes. It starts in middle age (35 to 50 years). There is no treatment. The patient slowly dies.

Parkinson's disease:

A problem with decay of nerves in the basal ganglia for which we do not know the cause is Parkinson's disease. The disease usually starts in old age. There is rigidity of some or all of the muscles of the body. There is also a tremor or shaking of the muscles. Sometimes it starts in one hand with a shaking that looks as if the patient is rolling pills. This is the "pill rolling" effect. There is some treatment for Parkinson's disease, but no real cure. The younger the disease starts, the worse it usually is.

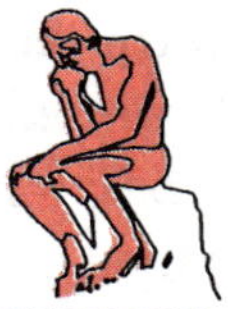

CONSIDER 26:9

HEMIBALLISMUS

Hemi means one-half. Ballismus means jumping about.

A girl was walking with her boyfriend. Suddenly her arm shot out and she knocked him out.

She was suffering from a disease called hemiballismus. The problem is thought to be caused by a small blood vessel stroke to the basal ganglia. The problem often goes away in one or two days.

What do you think of the girl's problem? What do you think her boyfriend thought?

****

SUMMARY
BASAL GANGLIA

The basal ganglia are masses of gray matter buried deep within the cerebrum. Interconnected, the basal ganglia have to do with fine movements such as writing and movements we do by habit such as tying shoes. Disease or injury to the basal ganglia causes jerky, stiff movements.

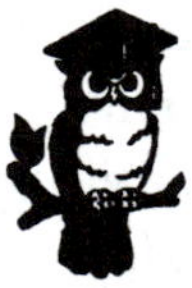

POP QUIZ:6

BASAL GANGLIA

True or False

1. The basal ganglia are buried deep within the cerebrum:
   T. F.

2. The basal ganglia have to do with sight and hearing:
   T. F.

3. The basal ganglia are involved primarily with curbing actions rather than starting actions:
   T. F.

DIENCEPHALON

"Dia" means between. The diencephalon ("be-tween-brain") develops as bulges on the neural tube above the developing brain stem.

As the diencephalon forms, so too do the two cerebral hemispheres. The hemispheres at first grow out and then back over the parts of the diencephalon. Finally, the hemispheres bury completely the diencephalon. Thus, just as with the basal ganglia, the diencephalon lies under and is completely covered by the cerebral hemispheres.

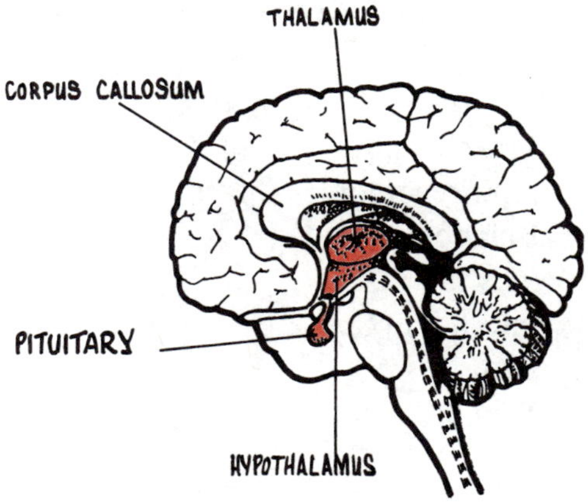

Fig. 28 Diencephalon

The diencephalon consists of two important structures: the **thalamus** and the **hypothalamus**. Connected to the diencephalon is another structure, the **pituitary gland**. Although the pituitary is only about two-fifths of an inch long, it is called the master gland of the body because it controls the functioning of many other glands. It also secretes a hormone that controls the growth rate of the body.

In our discussion of the diencephalon, we will also consider the "**limbic**" system. The limbic system is a group of glands and structures which play an important part in the regulation of body activities.

THALAMUS

"Thalamus" means inner chamber. The thalamus is about the size of an orange. It is mostly gray matter. It is just under the corpus callosum, the band of white matter connecting the two hemispheres of the cerebrum. From the thalamus, nerve fibers go to the cerebellum, spinal cord, cranial nerves, and the cerebral cortex.

The major function of the thalamus is to **relay impulses** from one part of the brain to another. The thalamus is also believed to play a role in the expression of **emotions**.

Through many tracts, the thalamus sends impulses to all areas of the cerebral cortex. The cortex, in turn, sends impulses back to the thalamus. It is impossible for the cerebral cortex to perform either sensory or motor functions without aid from the thalamus. But the thalamus can perform a few functions without the cerebral cortex. Therefore, it is probable that the thalamus plays at least some role in every cortical function.

Look at the thalamus as if it were the body's telephone system. Nerve endings under your skin receive impulses the same way a telephone does. These endings, like a telephone line, then send a message into your spinal cord . The message, such as pain from a tack, travels up the spinal cord and ends in the thalamus. The thalamus then sends the message on to the cerebral cortex.

Your brain answers the message and then sends an outgoing message that tells your body how to react.

SPINAL CORD	THALAMUS	CEREBRAL CORTEX
	Eyes..................*	....*
Muscle and joint receptors	..............*	....*
Balance organs in ears	..............*	....*
Internal organs	.............*	....*
Skin	..............*	....*
Tongue	..............*	....*
	Smell	....*

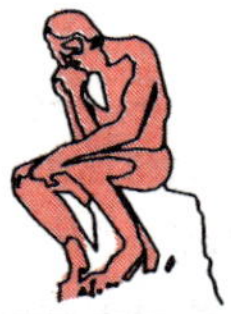

CONSIDER 26:10

THALAMUS

Atlanta, Georgia has a great airplane terminal. There is a saying, "Whether you are going to heaven or hell, you still have to change planes in Atlanta."

Think of the thalamus. Pain, temperature, touch, itching, all these sensations go to the cerebral cortex. In your cerebral cortex, your brain decides whether these sensations are good or bad. Then your cerebral cortex tells your body what to do.

But before any of these feelings reach your cerebral cortex they must all first stop in the thalamus. Do you think the thalamus is something like the air terminal in Atlanta?

There is one exception. The sense of smell does not stop in the thalamus. We will learn of that later.

****

HYPOTHALAMUS

"Hypo" means below or beneath. Below the thalamus, near the middle of the base of the brain, lies the **hypothalamus**. This peanut-sized mass of gray matter is an important part of the diencephalon.

METRONOME: A metronome is an instrument used to mark time by a repeated tick. Because it contains centers that control many internal activities, the hypothalamus is often called the **metronome of the body**.

The hypothalamus works with the autonomic (involuntary) nervous system to regulate various functions in the body. These include the heartbeat, blood pressure, pulse rate, body temperature, perspiration, sexual drive, blood sugar level, and body metabolism.

When a surgeon operates in the region of the hypothalamus, he must be careful. Just to pull on the tissue near the hypothalamus may cause changes in the heart rate, blood pressure, body temperature, etc.. As many as forty percent of the patients may die during surgery.

FIGHT OR FLIGHT: Special areas of the hypothalamus receive information about the blood pressure. They then send messages that help to adjust the blood pressure and heartbeat rate (pulse) to meet the body's needs.

If there is danger, the hypothalamus alerts the body. It makes the heart beat faster, sends more sugar into the blood (for energy), and increases the supply of the chemicals that make blood clot (in case you are injured and bleeding).

It also stops the digestive processes. This conserves energy for the muscles (in case you have to fight or run away). This is why, when you are frightened, you have a dry mouth.

REGULATION: The hypothalamus is the regulatory center for the production and release of many chemical substances (hormones). These hormones circulate in the blood. They control growth, development and many chemical reactions that occur in every cell of the body (metabolism). Its nerve cells control secretions, movement of the intestine, or stimulation of the pituitary gland.

EMOTIONS: This small island of gray matter is the source of such old feelings as anger, fear, hunger, thirst, and envy. When you are mad, the muscles that twist your face are probably controlled by the hypothalamus.

THERMOSTAT: One of the most important jobs of the hypothalamus is to control the body's temperature. As the body's "thermostat," the hypothalamus gets messages from heat cells in the skin. It measures the temperature of the blood passing through the brain. If you are too warm, the hypothalamus causes the capillaries in your skin to enlarge so your blood can cool. It may cause you to sweat and pant.

If you are cold, the hypothalamus causes blood vessels in the skin to close down. This cuts heat loss from the surface and saves it for vital organs such as your heart. You look blue and may shiver. If you were an animal or a bird, the hypothalamus would cause your hair or feathers to fluff up to help keep you warm.

APPESTAT: Another control center in the hypothalamus acts as a sort of "appestat," regulating the amount of food you eat. Actually, there are two separate control centers: a hunger center, which stimulates eating, and a satiety center, which gives a sensation of fullness.

A drop in glucose and other food materials in the blood triggers the hunger center. The satiety center responds to hormones that are released from the intestines while you are digesting the food from a meal. These controls do not seem to work properly in people who are overweight.

SLEEP CENTER: The sleep center is also thought to be in the hypothalamus. In the back part (posterior) of the hypothalamus is a "wakefulness" center, while in the front part (anterior) of the hypothalamus is an area dealing with sleep.

If the wakefulness center is stimulated with an electrical shock, the body sends out signals to the body telling it to wake up or stay awake.

The opposite is true with the sleep center. Stimulation here will put you to sleep.

PITUITARY GLAND

Pituitary means "mucous." This, because at one time the pituitary was thought to secrete a mucous like substance in the back of the throat. The pituitary is also called the hypophysis. "Hypophysis" means undergrowth. This, because of its attachment to the hypothalamus.

The pituitary is really two glands, an anterior or front lobe and a posterior or back lobe. The front lobe comes from the roof of the throat (pharynx). The back lobe falls down from the base of the brain and is connected by a stalk of nerves to the hypothalamus.

The pituitary is about two-fifths of an inch long. In the past, it was called the master gland of the body because it controls many other glands. Now, it is felt that this name is incorrect. Rather than being a master, the pituitary is, in many ways, the slave of the hypothalamus. It takes its orders from above and then passes them on to other glands.

SENTINEL GLAND: The front lobe of the pituitary greatly affects many other glands of the body. Therefore, it is often called the "**sentinel gland**."

Six important hormones that come from the front lobe of the pituitary are **thyrotrophic** hormone, **growth** hormone, **adrenocorticotrophic** hormone, **follicle stimulating** hormone, **luteinizing** hormone, and **luteotrophic** hormone.

Thyrotrophic hormone acts on the thyroid gland. Too much thyrotrophic hormone may cause your eyes to bulge.

Growth hormone affects all the cells of the body. If there is too much growth hormone secreted early in life, the victim could become an eight-foot giant. Later in life, if too much growth hormone is secreted, the victim won't get taller, but his hands and face may grow long. This condition is called acromegaly. Acro means extremity. Megaly means big.

Adrenocorticotrophic hormone acts on the small gland on top of each kidney called the adrenal gland. Ad means to. Ren means kidney.

These hormones regulate the use (metabolism) of carbohydrate, fat and protein. Too much of this hormone may result in obesity, too much hair, muscular development, and early sexuality. Older women with this problem may develop a deep voice and a moustache.

Gonadotrophic hormones: Gonadotrophic hormones are those hormones that effect the female ovaries and the male testicles. The front lobe of the pituitary secretes three of these hormones: follicle-stimulating hormone, luteinizing hormone, and luteotrophic hormone.

These hormones are secreted in only a small amount in the growing child. For unknown reasons, shortly before the child reaches puberty the pituitary begins to secrete large quantities of these hormones.

In the female, the secretion of these hormones causes the cycle of ovulation and menstruation. In the male, these hormones cause the growth of the testes, the formation of sperm, and the secretion of the male sex hormone, testosterone.

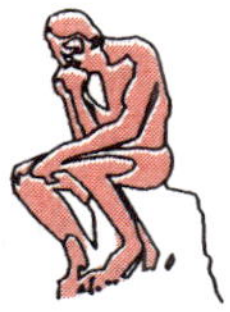

CONSIDER 26:11
LINCOLN

Some tumors of the pituitary gland result in overgrowth of the skeleton as in the condition acromegaly. The most common finding of acromegaly is overgrowth of the hands and feet. These changes take place gradually.

In addition to overgrowth of the hands and feet, the size of the skull increases and there is an overgrowth of facial hair. The lower jaw protrudes and there is widening of the spaces between the teeth. The tongue, lips, and nose are enlarged.

Considering the changes in his appearance over the years, some think that Abraham Lincoln may have suffered from acromegaly. What do you think?

****

ABNORMALITIES OF THE FRONT LOBE OF THE PITUITARY GLAND

Panhypopituitarism: Pan means all. Hypo means low. Panhypopituitarism means decreased secretion of all the frontal pituitary hormones. Here are some things which such victims may suffer from:

Dwarfism: There are several types of dwarfism. Those caused by a lack of secretion of pituitary hormones are Lorain dwarfs. The body of this dwarf develops in normal proportion but the rate of development is greatly decreased. A child of 10 may have the bodily development of one 4 or 5. At 20 he may have the development of a child of 7. The Lorain dwarf does not pass through puberty and does not develop adult sexual functions.

Senile type of dwarfism: Occasionally a child develops normally up until a certain age and suddenly his pituitary is destroyed by a tumor, disease, or blocked artery. When this happens, there is little further growth because of lack of growth hormone. No sexual functions begin; he loses his appetite and begins to look like a wrinkled old man. The skin is so wrinkled that a 10 year old boy may look like he is 80. A form of this is "progeria." Pro means before. Geras means old age.

Panhypopituitarism in the adult: Tumors or shock to the pituitary gland from a blood clot after a woman delivers a baby may cause hypopituitarism. A victim of this disease will always feel tired. She will gain weight and have no interest in sexual function.

Sometimes, rather than gain weight, a victim of panhypopituitarism will lose her appetite (anorexia). She gets thin and looks like the senile dwarf we described above. Without treatment, she will die in 6 months to a year.

BACK LOBE: The main function of the back lobe of the pituitary has to do with control of urine. It secretes a hormone called antidiuretic hormone that helps the body control fluids.

Without antidiuretic hormone, a victim will develop the condition called diabetes insipidus. Diabetes means to go through. Insipidus means not wise. In this condition, the victim will excrete 10 or 15 times the normal amount of daily urine. He will quickly become dried out. A victim of this condition can be treated by snorting powdered posterior pituitary extract into his nose. Don't confuse diabetes insipidus with the much more common disease, diabetes mellitus, which has to do with sugar metabolism, and for which people take insulin.

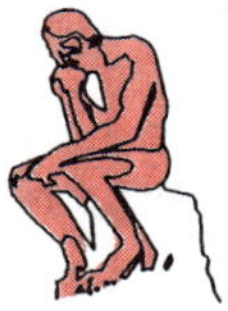

CONSIDER 26:12
THE IRISH GIANT

We have been studying the pituitary gland and its effect on the body. Consider a famous victim afflicted with a tumor of the anterior lobe of the pituitary gland, O'Brien or Byrne, **the Irish Giant.**

At the time of his death in 1783 at the age of twenty-two, O'Brien was 8 feet 4 inches tall. Pituitary giants do not live very long. This fact was known by a famous doctor of the time, John Hunter. Hunter was a collector of medical curiosities, particularly skeletons. He much wanted O'Brien's skeleton for his collection.

For his part, O'Brien certainly did not want his remains boiled in Hunter's kettle. For this reason, O'Brien moved often. But alas, soon up would pop Hunter.

Finally when O'Brien was ready to die, he paid some fishermen to take his body, after his death, out in the middle of the Irish Channel and sink it with heavy weights. Hunter found out about this and paid the fishermen even more to deliver O'Brien's body to him. It is said he paid 500 pounds for the body which, for the time, was a very large amount of money.

The skeleton, along with Hunter's kettle, is at the Museum of the Royal College of Surgeons in London. It measures 92 3/4 inches. It is exhibited alongside that of Caroline Crachami, the Sicilian dwarf, who was exhibited as an Italian princess in London in 1824. She did not grow after birth and died at the age of nine.

Don't you feel lucky that John Hunter is not your doctor?

****

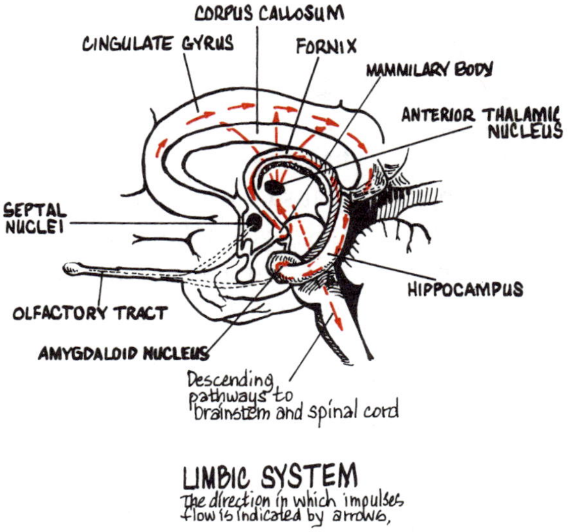

Fig. 29 Limbic System

LIMBIC SYSTEM

During evolution, man's brain evolved from a reptile's to a mammal's. The first part of the mammalian brain was the **limbic** system. Limbic means margin or edge. The limbic system is a ring of gray matter at the base of the cerebral cortex.

HIPPOCAMPUS: With some parts of the limbic system, such as the cingulate gyrus and parts of the hypothalamus, you are already familiar. Others are new, the most important being the **hippocampus**.

Hippocampus means "seahorse," which is what the ancient Greeks thought it looked like. To us, it resembles more a large bean pod.

RHINENCEPHALON: The limbic system, including the hippocampus, used to be called the rhinencephalon. Rhinencephalon means nose brain.

Lower mammals, such as mice, have a highly developed limbic system, which is closely associated with their sense of smell. The nerve by which we smell (olfactory) is, in reality, not a nerve at all. It is a projection of the brain with its base in the hippocampus.

The name rhinencephalon was changed to limbic system when it was found that it was much more important than had been thought. The limbic system is now felt to be the seat of **emotions**, as well as **smell**, **taste** and **sexual behavior**.

Paul MacLean, with the National Institute of Mental Health, has done much to define the limbic system. He feels that the close relationship of oral and genital functions in this part of the brain is due to the olfactory (smell) sense which, dating far back in evolution, plays an important part in both feeding and mating. The findings are relevant to oral-sexual displays in feeding, mating, and aggressive and violent behavior.

The limbic system gives us emotions. It lets us feel hope and enthusiasm. If there are setbacks, it allows us to feel despair. This, even though the setback may be due to a missed meal, a lost love, or a sense of danger.

The limbic system brings the setback to the attention of other parts of the cerebral cortex. The brain can then take steps to lessen the hurt.

AMYGDALA: The **amygdala** is another important part of the limbic system. Amygdala means almond, this because of its shape. This small mass of gray matter is the "window" through which you see your place in the world. The amygdala is also important in seeing and hearing.

If parts of the limbic system are destroyed, an animal may lose much of its personality. It may mate and have young, but then show no interest in the offspring.

If parts of the limbic system are stimulated, say by a small charge of electricity, an animal may feel intense pleasure. So much so, that if allowed to stimulate his brain at will by pressing a button, he will press the button until he falls over exhausted. Other parts of the limbic system when stimulated may cause pain or feelings of great sadness.

Some people who have had epileptic seizures involving the limbic system have described great joy. They wake up feeling that they have discovered the secret of all knowledge and everlasting happiness. They may be wrong, but to them it makes no difference, they have discovered the truth.

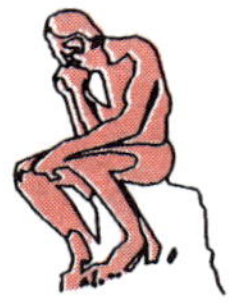

CONSIDER 26:13

THE TRIUNE BRAIN

What It Is

Triune means trinity or three in one. We have mentioned Doctor Paul MacLean with the National Institute of Mental Health and his work with the limbic system. Doctor MacLean coined the term "triune brain." It is a term he uses to describe the evolution of our brain. It means that, when we think, we are using three different brain mechanisms: two old brains and one new brain. And the bad part of it is that the two older brains can't talk.

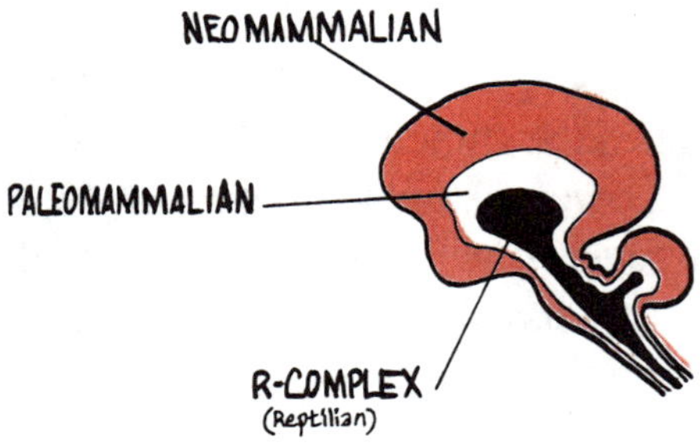

Fig. 30 Triune Brain

Their Names

The oldest brain is called the "R-complex." The next oldest brain is the "paleomammalian." With paleo meaning ancient, and mammalian meaning mammal, which is what we are. The next brain is the neomammalian, with neo meaning new.

Where They Come From

The R-complex comes from our earliest ancestors, the reptiles or lizards. This part of the brain is concerned with aggression, defense of territory, foraging, hunting and mating.

Two hundred million years ago we became little mammals and developed the paleomammalian brain. With this we began to recognize children that we cared for. We showed nursing traits, play, and the pain of separation from our offspring, hope, enthusiasm and despair.

Finally we developed the neomammalian brain. This is the large frontal lobes that correspond to our foreheads. This area is the most developed in man.

With the neomammalian brain comes feelings for others and a sense of consciousness. Also, there is an appreciation that present actions may have consequences down the road.

So What?

Some drugs (including alcohol) attack the brain from above downward. That is, the drug attacks first the higher centers of the brain. People on these drugs may show the wide stance, stiff-gaited and aggressive, puffed up behavior of lizards. Many violent criminals show damage to both the neomammalian and paleomammalian parts of the brain.

Some geniuses, such as Einstein, are mostly loners. They show little of the socialization characteristic of the neomammalian brain.

****

SUMMARY
DIENCEPHALON

The diencephalon is that portion of the brain **between** the cerebrum and the midbrain. Three important structures associated with the diencephalon are the thalamus, hypothalamus and the pea-shaped pituitary (hypophysis).

The orange-sized thalamus relays impulses from one part of the brain to another. Except the sense of smell, all functions between the brain and other parts of the body pass through the thalamus.

The peanut-sized hypothalamus is important in the regulation of bodily functions. It exerts major control over the heartbeat, blood pressure, pulse rate, temperature, perspiration, sex drive, metabolism and blood sugar level.

The hypothalamus is also important in controlling the release of hormones and regulating the appetite. Our sleep center is in the hypothalamus.

The small pituitary gland is important for hormone production. The front lobe of the pituitary, also called the "sentinel gland," has to do with growth and reproduction. Disease of the front lobe of the pituitary gland can result in dwarfism or gigantism. The back lobe of the pituitary gland helps control urine production.

The limbic system is made up of parts which were originally our ancient brain. The limbic system is felt to be the seat of emotions, as well as taste and sexual behavior.

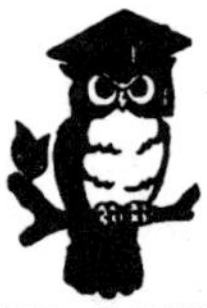

POP QUIZ:7
DIENCEPHALON

Circle the correct answer

1. The diencephalon is part of:
   A. forebrain B. midbrain C. hindbrain

2. Two structures in the diencephalon are the hypothalamus and the:
   A. corpus callosum B. thalamus C. amygdala

3. The thalamus plays a part in all cortical functions except:
   A. sight B. sound C. smell D. taste

4. The hypothalamus has been called the body's:
   A. eyes B. ears C. nose D. metronome

5. The hypothalamus helps control:
   A. digestion B. appetite C. sleep
   D. all of the above

6. The pituitary gland is divided into how many lobes:
   A. one B. two C. three D. four

True or False

7. The pituitary is important in hormone secretion:
   T. F.

8. Abnormality of the pituitary gland may lead to gigantism:
   T. F.

9. Abnormality of the pituitary gland may lead to dwarfism:
   T. F.

10. The limbic system is felt to be the most primitive part of our brain:
    T. F.

MIDBRAIN (MESENCEPHALON)

The midbrain is about an inch square. It is the narrowest portion of the brain. It is at the top of the brain stem just under the thalamus. It is surrounded by the two cerebral hemispheres.

All impulses traveling to or from the cerebrum and diencephalon must pass through the midbrain. For this reason, it is called the bottleneck of the brain.

The midbrain aids in regulating alertness. It also has to do with balance and posture. It has some centers concerned with hearing, vision, eye movement and control of reactions such as the contraction of the pupil in bright light.

HINDBRAIN (RHOMBENCEPHALON)

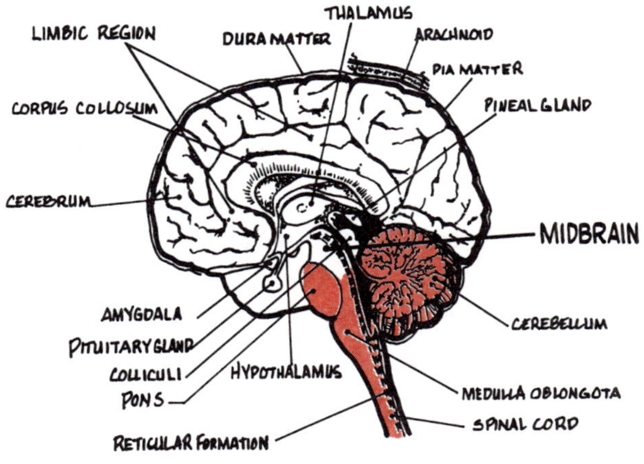

Fig. 31 Hindbrain

Evolution means a change from a simple state into one more complex. The brain of man evolved from simple animals into the complex brain of today. The first part of our brains came from those like a lizards. This is the hindbrain.

Now lizards don't talk, read books, or wear funny hats, because they have lizard brains and not human brains. Lizards do lizard things, and because our brains are also part lizard brains, we too do lizard things.

So the question is, "What does our hindbrain enable us to do that lizards do?" The answer, "Many things." In fact, with only our hindbrain, we could get along quite well. Not very well, but quite well.

Things our hind brain enables us to do: it controls the rate of heartbeat, and our breathing. It maintains our blood pressure and lets us swallow. It allows us to walk and move our hand to our mouth.

According to Dr. MacLean, if you are a lizard with only a hindbrain, this may be your daily routine: You get up in the morning and emerge from your den. Cautiously you look around for enemies. Feeling safe, you lie in the sun for a while to warm up (you have no internal temperature regulation). Then you defecate, after which you go hunting, eat, take a nap, run around a little, lie in the sun some more and then go home.

If there are other lizards in the area, you may put on your act. You will puff up to show what a big strong guy you are and fight to protect your territory. If the other lizard is bigger, tougher, or a better bluffer, you may bow your head and slink away. You may mate.

A bad thing about having only a lizard brain is that you cannot adjust to new situations. If, when you get home, a rock has rolled over the opening to your den, it may take you a long time to figure out the problem, still longer to decide what to do about it. And, of course, you are unable to call for help.

If, by some chance, you could call for help, and your mother heard, that would be bad news. Your mother, also having a lizard brain, would have no centers for emotion, and so she would eat you.

CEREBELLUM: The hind brain consists of the cerebellum and the brain stem. First we will consider the cerebellum.

We know that "cerebrum" means brain. With the diminutive suffix "ellum" added to the end, "**cerebellum**" means little brain.

The cerebellum is behind the brain stem and underneath the occipital lobes of the cerebrum. It looks like two loosely rolled balls of twine. These two lobes are connected in the middle by another lobe which, because of its cross-wise furrows and ridges, is called the **worm** (vermiform process) .

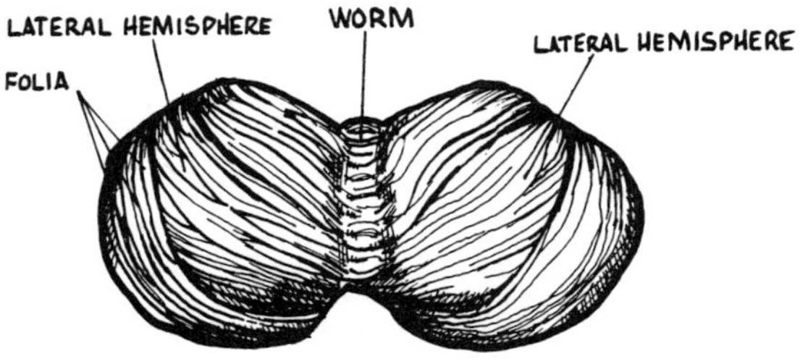

Fig. 32 Cerebellum

The cerebellum is the size of an orange and is about ten percent of the brain's weight. Like the cerebrum, the surface of the cerebellum is gray matter and the deeper portion is white matter. The gray matter of the cerebellum is darker than that of the cerebrum.

Its surface is patterned with grooves and ridges but, unlike the cerebrum, it has no gyri and sulci. Instead, the cerebellum is made up of folds called **folia** (leaf). Each folia controls a different part of the body.

If the cerebellum is traced upwards from fish through amphibians and reptiles to birds, it will be seen that the cerebellum varies greatly in size. Those creatures that creep and crawl have small cerebellums. Great swimmers and flyers have large cerebellums. This, because of the effect of the cerebellum on muscles, particularly those dealing with coordination and movement.

The cerebellum receives fibers from the cerebral cortex above and from the spinal cord below. Acting together with the rest of the brain, the cerebellum controls your **posture** and **balance**. It provides smooth cooperation between mind and muscle.

If the cerebellum is touched with an electric current, inhibition occurs. By inhibition is meant that if you are holding your arm out and your cerebellum is stimulated then your arm would suddenly fall to your side. The muscles causing your arm to extend are inhibited. They are stopped.

People whose cerebellums have been damaged cannot move properly. If they try to reach out to something, they reach too far before they can stop themselves. If they move an arm or leg very rapidly, they may lose track of exactly where it is . They find it difficult to keep their balance when they walk or run. They may stagger and feel dizzy.

With a damaged cerebellum, if you tried to write, your letters would stray all over the paper. If you tried to sew, you would be always sticking yourself.

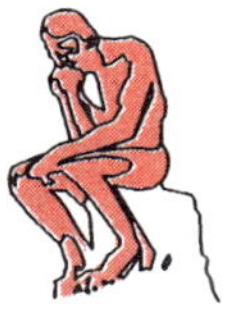

CONSIDER 26:14

THREE SIGNS

There are three signs, well known to medical students, which may show damage to the cerebellum. These are Romberg's sign, Stewart-Holmes' sign and Past Pointing.

ROMBERG'S SIGN

In Romberg's sign, while standing, when the patient with cerebellar disease is asked to close his eyes, he will stagger and may fall over.

STEWART-HOLMES' SIGN

In Stewart-Holmes sign, if you should hold your hand up and block the fist of the patient, then you suddenly moved your hand, the patient's fist would shoot out and he couldn't stop it.

What do you think of these two signs? They are named after the doctors who first described them.

PAST POINTING

Another sign of cerebellar disease is "past-pointing." In this test, the patient stands with eyes closed and arms outstretched. He is asked to touch his nose with his right thumb. In cerebellar disease, the patient will usually miss his nose and may poke himself in the eye. This may also be seen in acute alcoholism. In fact, in alcoholism the patient may even miss his nose with his eyes open.

****

BRAIN STEM

The second major division of the hindbrain is the brain stem. We divide the brain stem into three parts: **Pons, Medulla Oblongata** and **Reticular Activating System**.

PONS

Pons means bridge. This bulb-shaped mass of mostly white matter forms a bridge between the two sides of the cerebellum, and also connects the cerebrum above and the medulla oblongata below.

Through this passageway pass fibers between the medulla, the cerebrum, and the cerebellum. What gray matter the pons has is important because cranial nerves 3,4,5,6,7 and 8 arise from within it. We will soon study the cranial nerves.

MEDULLA OBLONGATA

Medulla means fat, grease or like the marrow of bone. Other meanings might be the essence or pith of a substance. A way of saying this is that the medulla is the "true grit" of the brain. Oblongata means long.

The medulla oblongata is the oldest part of your brain. It is formed by the folding of body cells. Then it is pushed up into your head by the growth of the rest of the body.

This first part of the brain grows out of the spinal cord. There cannot be seen any definite dividing line between the medulla and the spinal cord. Once in the skull, the medulla enlarges into a funnel or triangular shape. It is sometimes called "the spinal bulb." It is only about an inch long and three quarters of an inch wide.

From the day you are born until you die, the medulla keeps a day-and-night vigil over the automatic movements inside your body. These are heartbeat, breathing, swallowing, and blood pressure.

Because the medulla controls breathing and the heart beat, a karate chop to the back of the neck can bring instant unconsciousness or even death. From the medulla, several cranial nerves supply the muscles of the head and neck, including the muscles we use to speak and to swallow.

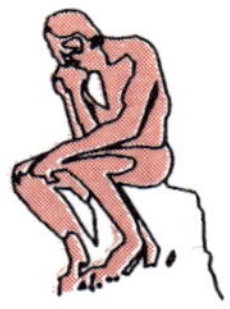

CONSIDER 26:15

ONDINE'S CURSE

Ondine's Curse is a rare sleep problem of children in which they quit breathing when they sleep. The problem is at the base of the brain. Because of some unknown disorder of the sleep center in the hindbrain, when the child is asleep, the brain does not tell him to breathe. As a result, most of these children die.

Now, a few children who have the problem quickly diagnosed can survive. They are kept on artificial respirators until the condition is overcome. Sometimes the name "Ondine's Curse" is given to other problems where, when asleep, the sufferer either quits breathing or has trouble breathing.

The name Ondine's Curse comes from an old German legend. "Ondine" comes from the Latin word "Undine," meaning wave.

Undine was a water spirit. She was the daughter of the water prince of the Mediterranean. She would get a soul if she married a mortal man.

Undine, a child of three, was coming from a lake when she was found by a fisherman and his wife, who had lost their own daughter of the same age by drowning. The couple brought up the child who, when she was 18, fell in love with a lost traveler. The traveler was a knight, Count Huldbrand, who had been sent on a quest by his fair lady, Bertalda.

Undine won the count's affections, and they were married. Now, with her newly acquired soul which bestowed meekness, loving-kindness, and thoughtfulness she went with her count back to the castle where Bertalda still awaited the Count's return.

There occurred a love triangle in which Bertalda again became the favorite. When the three were on a ship in the Danube, the arm of a water spirit arose and snatched a necklace from Bertalda. Undine drew from the water an even more beautiful necklace.

Huldbrand grew mad at the water spirits, including his wife, and cursed her. He forgot that he had been told never to curse his wife near the water. As a penalty, Undine had to go back into the water from which she had come.

Following Undine's presumed death, Huldbrand and Bertalda decided to marry. This, in spite of a dream in which Huldbrand had been warned by the water spirits that if he remarried he would die. After the marriage, Bertalda reopened an old fountain. Out of the waters came Undine to remind Huldbrand of the fate of a faithless husband. Repentant, he died with her kiss on his lips.

What do you think of Ondine's Curse, both the disease and the myth? Does it reinforce in your mind how important one little area of your brain might be?

****

RETICULAR ACTIVATING SYSTEM

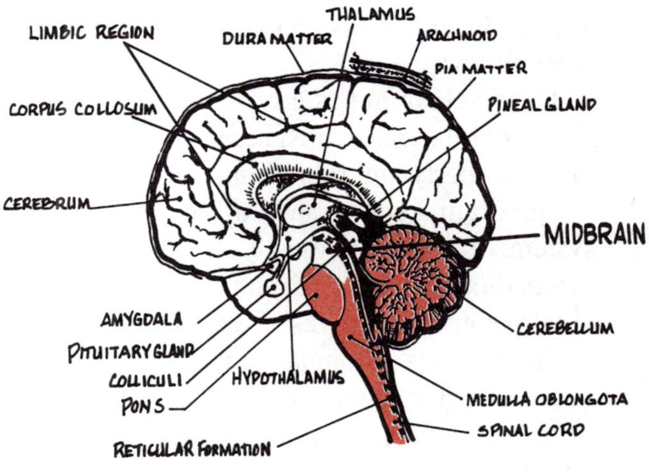

Fig. 33 Cross Section Of Brain

Reticulum means a net. The reticular activating system is a mass of gray matter in the form of a sheath or net that goes all the way from the spinal cord into the thalamus, hypothalamus, cerebellum and the cortex.

The reticular activating system is that group of neurons that "brings it all together." It is the main **uniting center** for all the brain's activities and the **center of consciousness**.

The reticular activating system decides what information is important enough to report to the higher portions of the brain. You are aware of only that information that your reticular activating system wants your cerebrum to receive.

If you are excited, your reticular activating system may cause your heart to beat faster without your being aware of what is happening. When it is time for you to sleep, your reticular activating system shuts down the impulses going to your brain so that you may rest. You no longer hear traffic outside or the clock ticking. However, if there is the scent of smoke, your reticular activating system may send an urgent message to your brain so that you awake.

If you are studying in a crowded room, your reticular activating system may shut out all noise. Then you may concentrate on your work. However, if your sweetheart should whisper to you, your reticular activating system would shout, "Hey! This is important." Your eyes would pop open, and you would turn toward the whisper.

SUMMARY
MIDBRAIN & HINDBRAIN

The midbrain is between the diencephalon and the hindbrain. The midbrain aids in regulating alertness. It helps control pupil size to bright light and is important in preserving balance.

In terms of evolution, the hindbrain or rhombencephalon is the oldest part of our brains. It is made up of the cerebellum and brain stem . If we possessed only a hindbrain, we would function in a most primitive manner like a lizard.

The cerebellum, the size of an orange, helps to control balance. Those animals that swim and fly have larger cerebellums than animals which creep or crawl. Infants have small cerebellums.

The cerebellum has grooves which separate it into leafs or folia. It is divided into three lobes, two lateral hemispheres and the worm. People with damaged cerebellums cannot move properly and fall often.

The brain stem is made up of the pons, medulla oblongata and the reticular activating system. The pons is mostly white matter, relaying messages between the two sides of the cerebellum and the cerebrum above and medulla oblongata below. It has a small amount of gray matter which gives rise to several cranial nerves.

The medulla oblongata is the oldest part of the brain. The medulla maintains vigil over autonomic movements inside the body such as heartbeat and respiration.

The reticular activating system is a sheath of gray matter which goes from the spinal cord into the cerebral cortex. It is the main uniting system for all the brain's activities. It filters out messages which it does not feel need immediate attention.

POP QUIZ:8
MIDBRAIN & HINDBRAIN

True or False

1. The midbrain is sometimes called the "bottleneck" of the brain:
   T. F.

2. The midbrain may help control the contraction of the pupil in bright light:
   T. F.

3. Boys who behave like lizards may be using only their hindbrain:
   T. F.

4. The middle lobe of the cerebellum is called the maggot:
   T. F.

5. The cerebellum is made up of partitions called folia:
   T. F.

6. Each folia serves several parts of the body:
   T. F.

7. With a damaged cerebellum you will walk a straight line:
   T. F.

8. Considering their size, snails and infants have very large cerebellums:
   T. F.

9. The pons and medulla oblongata are parts of the brain stem:
   T. F.

10. The pons is a bridge between the two cerebellar hemispheres:
    T. F.

11. The medulla oblongata is the oldest part of your brain:
    T. F.

12. Damage to the medulla oblongata may result in instant death:
    T. F.

13. A person with a malfunctioning respiratory section of the medulla oblongata may stop breathing when he falls asleep:
    T. F.

14. The reticular activating system is a net of gray matter beginning in the thalamus and ending in the cerebrum:
    T. F.

15. The reticular activating system may filter out messages coming to your brain which it does not feel need immediate attention:
T. F.

CRANIAL NERVES

Cranium means the upper part of the head. The cranial nerves are twelve nerves that arise from the brain and emerge through openings (**foramina**) of the skull. They are numbered according to the order in which they pass through the dura mater at the base of the skull. They are also given names as to the organ or function they serve.

Some cranial nerves are purely sensory, some entirely motor, and others mixed. The cranial nerves are connected to some part of the surface of the brain. But always, their fibers can be traced deeply into the brain to some special center of gray matter termed a nucleus. This is their deep or real origin.

Before studying the cranial nerves, it may be wise to review some terms we use when speaking of nerves. An "afferent" nerve is one that carries a message to the brain. An "efferent" nerve is one that carries a message away from the brain.

A "sensory" nerve is the same as an afferent nerve. A sensory nerve carries a message from a sense organ, such as the ear, to the brain. A "motor" nerve is often the same as an efferent nerve. A motor nerve goes from the brain to a part, such as a muscle, to make it move or a salivary gland to make it produce mucous (spit).

OLFACTORY NERVE

The first cranial nerve is the olfactory nerve. This is not just one nerve, but about twenty. They come off the olfactory bulb, which is an oval mass of grayish color under the frontal lobe of the brain. The olfactory nerves are really a forward projecting part of the brain.

The olfactory nerves are entirely afferent. They send messages deep within the brain.

In injuries to the head, the olfactory bulb may become separated from the olfactory nerves.

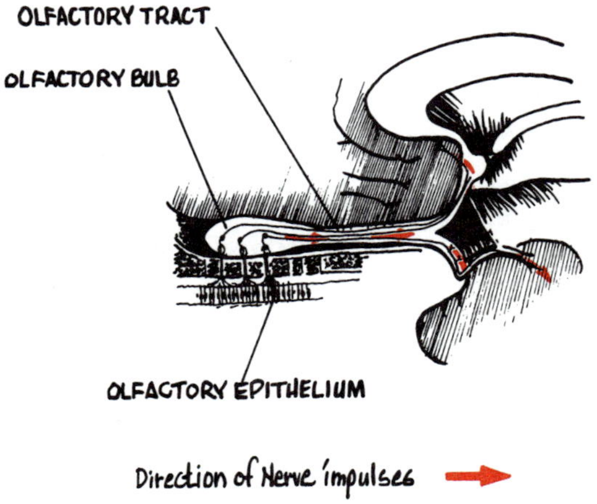

Fig. 34 Olfactory Nerve

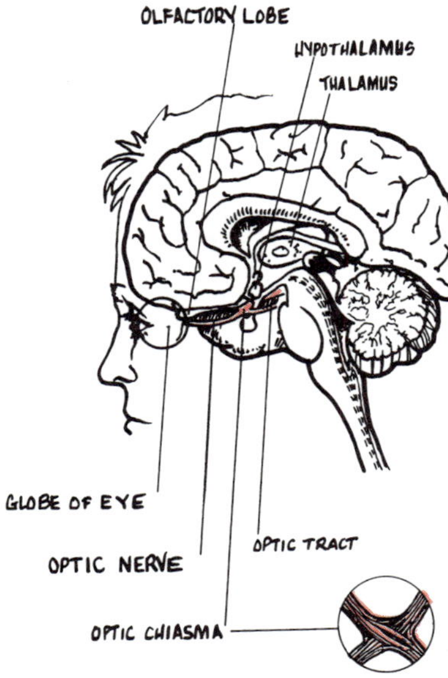

Fig. 35 Optic Nerve

This causes a loss of the sense of smell (anosmia). Because many foods give off odors which also excite the sense of **taste**, there may also be a loss of the sense of taste.

OPTIC NERVE

The second cranial nerve is the optic nerve. Like the olfactory nerve, the optic nerve is also a part of the brain. It serves the sense of **sight** and is mostly afferent.

The optic nerve fibers start from the back of the eye (retina). The nerves from each eye then enter the skull and meet at the optic **chiasma**. "Chiasma" means to mark with the letter X or a crossing.

At the chiasma, the fibers from the nose side of the eye cross to the other side of the brain. The fibers from the ear side of the eye do not cross. Thus, both sides of the brain receive some fibers from both eyes. As we have studied, the fibers then go to the thalamus. The optic nerve is subject to injury from many causes resulting in loss of vision.

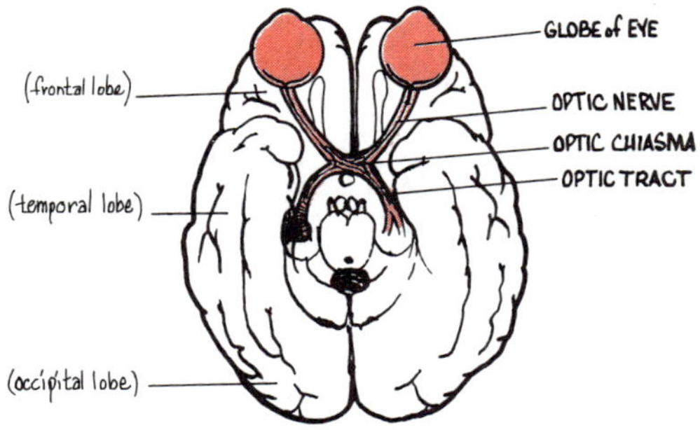

Fig. 36 Optic Tract

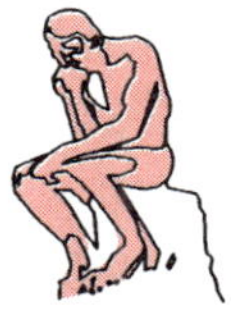

CONSIDER 26:16
ALCOHOL - TOBACCO AMBLYOPIA

An interesting condition is Alcohol-Tobacco Amblyopia. "Amblyopia" means dimness of vision. In this problem there is a color blindness in the central field of vision in both eyes.

This condition is seen most often in middle-aged or elderly males who smoke a pipe and drink large amounts of alcohol. If the condition has not gone too far, absolute withdrawal from all forms of alcohol and tobacco will result in improvement of vision.

****

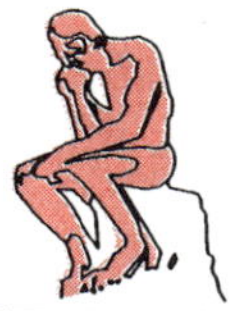

CONSIDER 26:17
A TRAGEDY

A young man was depressed. He thought he was a burden to his family. He put a gun to the side of his head and pulled the trigger.

The bullet went through his brain. The only damage it did was to completely cut the optic chiasma. From that day on he was blind.

Where on the diagram did the bullet pass? Do you feel that he was then more or less a burden to his family?

****

OCULOMOTOR, TROCHLEAR, AND ABDUCENS NERVES

The third, fourth and sixth cranial nerves will be studied together. All three have to do with **movement of the eyes**. Injury to the nuclei or nerves of these three nerves causes double vision, cross-eyes, and trouble moving the eyes.

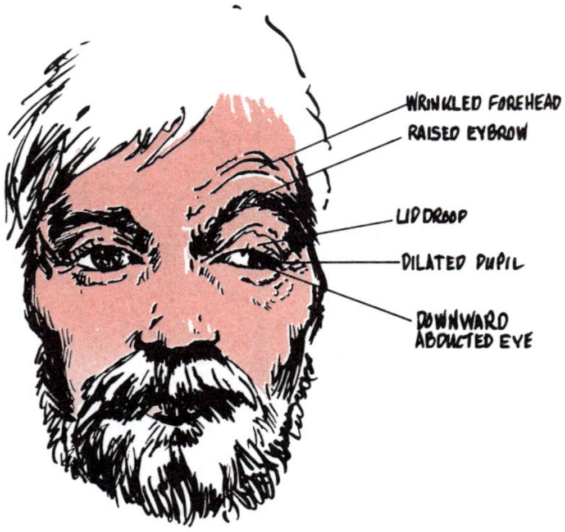

Fig. 37 Oculomotor Nerve Paralysis

OCULOMOTOR NERVE: Oculus means eye. Motor means mover. This nerve supplies some muscles of the eye, also the upper eye lid and the pupil.

Injury to the oculomotor nerve results in a falling of the upper eye lid. The victim's eye looks like that of a bloodhound. He cannot open his eye. The eyeball looks out and downward. The eye pupil is wide open (dilated) and does not close when a light is shined in it.

TROCHLEAR NERVE: Trochlear means pulley. The trochlear nerve is the smallest of the cranial nerves. It supplies one of the upper (superior) eye muscles.

Injury to the trochlear nerve causes the victim to lose the ability to turn his eye downward and outward. If he tries to look down and outward, this causes his other eye to be twisted inward so that he sees double. Thus, when he goes down hill or down stairs, he sees double and becomes dizzy.

ABDUCENS NERVE: The sixth cranial nerve is the abducens nerve. Abducens means drawing away from. The abducens nerve supplies a muscle that moves the eyeball outward.

Injury to the abducens nerve causes the victim to have cross-eyes with the eyeball turning in toward the nose. He has double vision. A fracture to the back of the head or base of the skull most often causes injury to this nerve. Increased pressure in the skull, such as from meningitis, may cause paralysis of the abducens nerve.

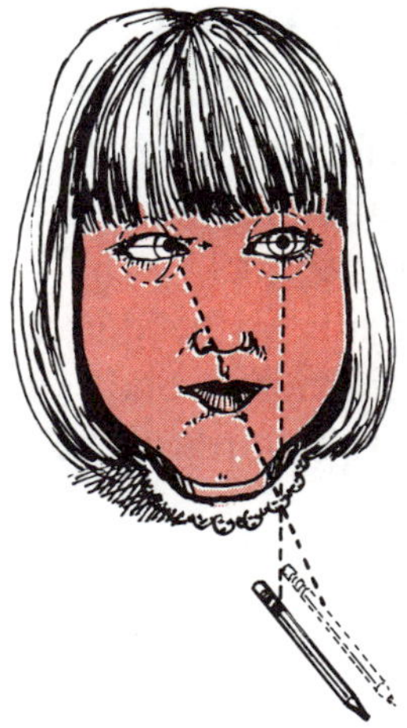

Fig. 38 Abducens Nerve Injury

TRIGEMINAL NERVE

The fifth cranial nerve is the trigeminal nerve. Trigeminal means three twins. It is called trigeminal because it has three main divisions: **ophthalmic**, **superior maxillary**, and **inferior maxillary**.

The trigeminal is the largest cranial nerve. It is the great sensory nerve of the head and face. It also is motor in supplying the muscles that have to do with chewing (mastication).

Injury to the trigeminal nerve makes a victim unable to chew. His jaw points to the side of the injury. Also, he has no sensation to his face. This means that he cannot feel a fly crawling on his nose or a pin sticking in his cheek. He does not know if he has something in his eye.

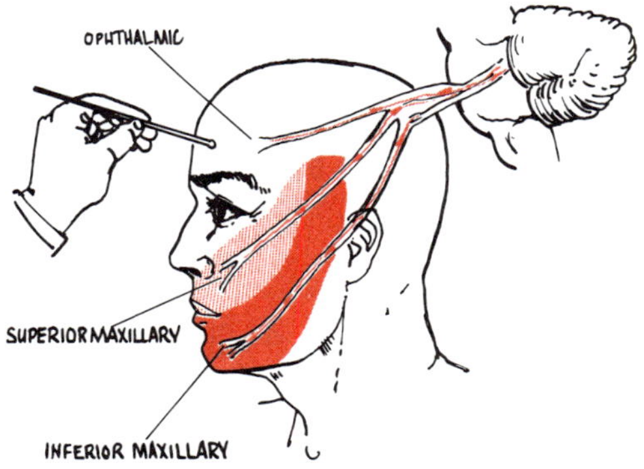

Fig. 39 Trigeminal Nerve

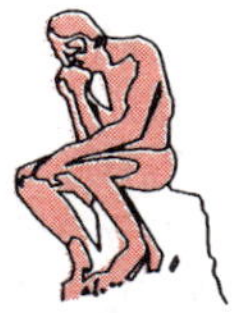

CONSIDER 26:18

TIC DOULOUREUX

A tic is a muscular spasm or contraction. Douloureux is French and means painful. This is a very painful condition of one of the sensory divisions of the trigeminal nerve. The victim with this condition experiences sharp, stabbing sensations to the face and jaw that come and go.

The cause of tic douloureux is not known. It may occur at any age, but is more common in middle or late life. Cases have been reported in children at the age of ten.

Attacks may occur many times a day, or several times a month. The searing, lightning-like jabs of pain may last a few seconds or several minutes. Between attacks, there is no pain, but the patient always fears that another attack might occur.

Treatment of tic douloureux is not good. Pain medication with even the strongest pain killers does not usually relieve the pain. Often the patient must have surgery to cut branches of the nerve.

****

FACIAL NERVE

The seventh cranial nerve is the facial nerve. This nerve is both motor and sensory. It supplies efferent fibers to the muscles of **facial expression**. It sends fibers to the cheek muscle, called the buccinator or trumpeters' muscle. It also sends fibers to the platysma muscle in the neck. The platysma is called the "shaver's muscle" because when a man shaves he tilts his head up and tenses the platysma which is just under the skin.

The facial nerve sends afferent or sensory fibers to the brain monitoring taste on the front (anterior) two-thirds of the tongue. Fracture to the head may often cause injury to the facial nerve.

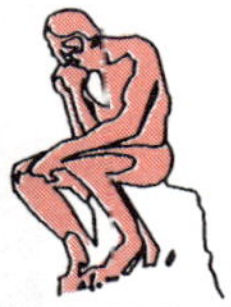

CONSIDER 26:19
BELL'S PALSY

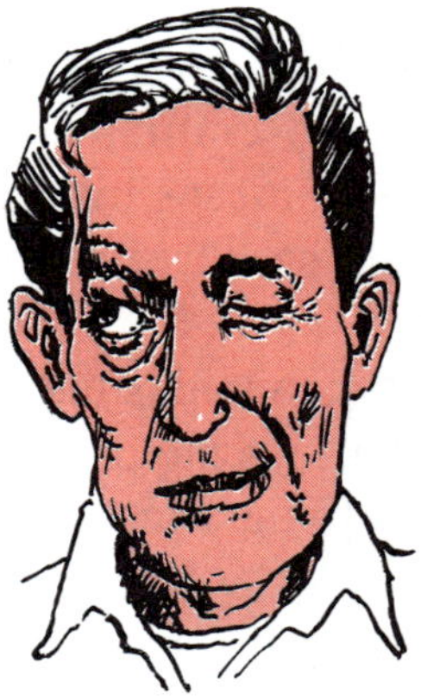

Fig. 40 Bell's Palsy
right side is paralyzed

The facial nerve is the most often paralyzed of any of the cranial nerves. One of the most common injuries to the facial nerve is Bell's Palsy.

In Bell's Palsy, the victim cannot wrinkle his forehead or close his eye. Because his lips on one side are paralyzed, he seems to be talking out of one side (the good) of his mouth. Because his buccinator muscle is paralyzed, when he tries to puff out his cheeks, air escapes out his mouth.

The cause of Bell's Palsy is not known. It is thought to be due to exposure to the cold.

Treatment also is not very good. Cortisone drugs may be helpful. Surgery is not usually recommended.

Fortunately, after a few weeks, most cases get better on their own. A few victims may have permanent partial or complete paralysis.

****

ACOUSTIC NERVE

The eighth cranial nerve is the acoustic nerve. The word acoustic relates to **hearing**.

The acoustic nerve has two branches: the **cochlear** which deals with **hearing** and the **vestibular** which deals with **balance**.

Cochlea means spiral. This pertains to the spiral, sea shell appearing, structure in our heads that monitors our hearing. A person with injury to the cochlear branch of the seventh nerve will have a hearing loss and ringing (tinnitus) in the ear.

Vestibule means entrance. This has to do with the entrance to three half circles (**semicircular canals**) on each side of the head. These canals oversee our balance. A person with damage to the vestibular division of the facial nerve will be dizzy.

A blow to the ear, such as with a cupped hand, may cause permanent hearing loss. Loud noises, such as gunfire or too loud "rock music," may also cause permanent hearing loss.

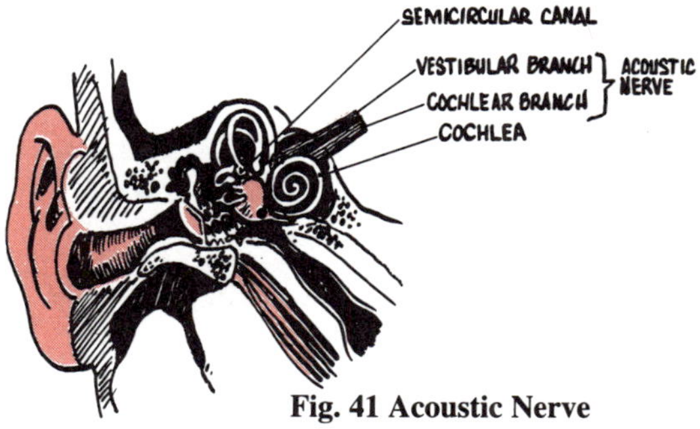

Fig. 41 Acoustic Nerve

GLOSSOPHARYNGEAL NERVE

The ninth cranial nerve is the glossopharyngeal nerve. Glosso means **tongue**. Pharyngeal has to do with the **mouth**. It is usually used to mean the back of the mouth. As the name implies, the glossopharyngeal nerve deals with the tongue and the back of the mouth.

The glossopharyngeal is the nerve of **taste** to the **back** (posterior) third of the **tongue**, and of **pain** to the back of the **throat**, **tonsils**, and **middle ear**. In addition, it has fibers that go to the salivary glands to monitor the amount of saliva in your mouth.

Sometimes when someone has his tonsils out and then eats, he will feel that he has an infection in his ear. This is because the glossopharyngeal nerve that supplies the tonsils also has fibers in the middle ear. The brain thinks that pain coming from where the tonsils were removed is coming from the ear.

GLOSSOPHARYNGEAL NEURALGIA: Glossopharyngeal neuralgia is like tic douloureux. Only, instead of the fifth nerve being involved, in this case it is the ninth cranial nerve which is inflamed.

Like tic douloureux, the cause of glossopharyngeal neuralgia is not known. Men in their forties and fifties are most frequently affected.

A person with this problem feels sharp stabbing pains in his throat, back of the tongue, and his ear. Swallowing or chewing sometimes causes an attack to occur. Because they are afraid to swallow, the victims of this disease sometimes do not eat and so become thin and weak.

Treatment of glossopharyngeal neuralgia is surgical. The nerve is cut while it is still inside the skull. The sufferer has immediate relief from his pain, and there are few side effects.

VAGUS NERVE

The tenth cranial nerve is the vagus nerve. Vagus means **wandering**. This is a good name for the tenth nerve because it has the widest distribution of the cranial nerves. Because it supplies the **lungs**, **heart**, **stomach**, and **intestines**, the tenth cranial nerve is also called the pneumogastric nerve.

The vagus has both motor and sensory fibers. It supplies the voice and lungs with motor and sensory fibers. It supplies the throat, oesophagus (food tube), stomach and heart with motor fibers.

One branch of the vagus nerve, the recurrent laryngeal nerve, arises in the chest. On the left side, it wraps around the large artery coming from the heart (aorta), then travels up the neck to supply the vocal cords (larynx). If someone has swelling of the aorta (aneurysm) or cancer in the chest or oesophagus, the first symptom he may have is paralysis of one of his vocal cords. His voice will be hoarse.

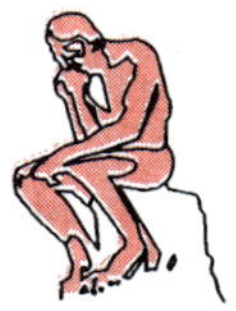

CONSIDER 26:20
ARNOLD'S NERVE

A small branch of the vagus nerve, "Arnold's nerve," goes to the ear canal. For this reason, someone with a bug in his ear or a child with an ear infection may have coughing fits.

A doctor was cleaning a patient's ear. She started to cough and said, "Excuse me." She thought it was her fault that she coughed. What do you think?

****

SPINAL ACCESSORY NERVE

The eleventh cranial nerve is the spinal accessory nerve. This is a motor nerve. The spinal portion of the nerve sends fibers to the **neck** (sternocleidomastoid) muscle. It also sends fibers to the large muscle of the **back** and neck called the trapezius. Trapezius means "a little table," or "table shaped."

The accessory portion of the spinal accessory nerve sends fibers along with the vagus nerve to the throat and voice box and the roof of the mouth.

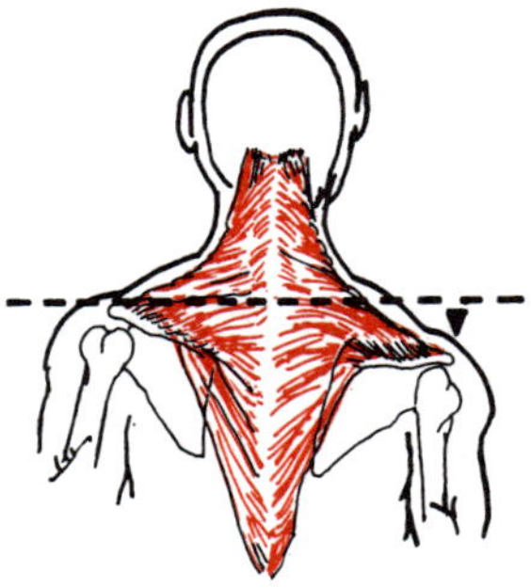

Fig. 42 Accessory Nerve Injury
right shoulder droop

Sometimes, in treating cases of throat cancer that has spread to the neck, it is necessary to cut the spinal accessory nerve. These patients end up with a drooping shoulder on the afflicted side.

HYPOGLOSSAL NERVE

The twelfth cranial nerve is the hypoglossal nerve. Hypoglossal means "under the tongue." This is a motor nerve to the **muscles of the tongue**.

A neck injury might harm the hypoglossal nerve. In this case, when the victim sticks out his tongue, the tongue will deviate toward the injured side.

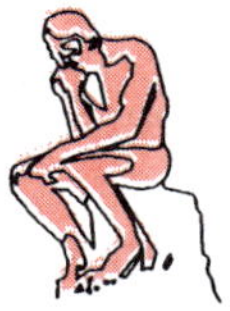

CONSIDER 26:21
ALCOHOLISM

Often in alcoholism, the hypoglossal nerve is irritated. In these cases, the patient's tongue seems to be jumping all over his mouth. A doctor, when looking in such a patient's mouth and seeing his tongue wiggling like a snake, might say, "You are going to have to quit drinking, Sam."

To this, Sam would reply, "How did you know I drank?" He would not know that his own tongue told on him.

****

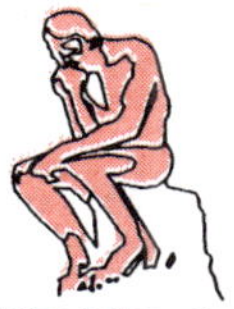

CONSIDER 26:22
A MNEMONIC

A mnemonic, pronounced knee-mahn-ick, is a device used to help memory. Medical students often use jingles as a mnemonic. One such jingle is the following: On Old Olympia's Towering Tops, A Fin And German Viewed Some Hops.

The first letter of each word in the jingle corresponds to cranial nerves one through twelve: Olfactory, Optic, Oculomotor, Trochlear, Trigeminal, Abducens, Facial, Auditory, Glossopharyngeal, Vagus, Spinal accessory, Hypoglossal.

What do you think of this mnemonic? You might want to make up mnemonics to help you in your studies.

****

SUMMARY
CRANIAL NERVES

We have twelve cranial nerves that arise from the brain and emerge through openings of the skull. The cranial nerves are numbered as to the order in which they pass through the dura mater at the base of the skull. They also have names indicating the organ or function that they serve.

The olfactory nerve serves the sense of smell. The optic nerve serves sight. Three nerves, oculomotor, trochlear and abducens, are responsible for eye movement.

The large trigeminal nerve is the sensory nerve of the face. It also supplies muscles involved in chewing.

If you should injure your facial nerve, you would be unable to smile or close your eye on the side of the injury. Also, you would be unable to taste things on the front two-thirds of your tongue.

The acoustic is the eighth cranial nerve. The cochlear branch of the eighth nerve has to do with hearing. If the vestibular branch of the acoustic nerve is injured, the patient may suffer from dizziness.

Glosso means tongue. Pharynx deals with the throat. The ninth cranial nerve is the glossopharyngeal nerve. This nerve supplies taste to the back of the tongue and pain to the back of the throat. In addition, it stimulates the salivary glands to produce mucous (spit).

Vagus means wandering. The long tenth nerve wanders from the brain to the ear, then to the throat. From the lungs it sends a nerve back up to the voice box (larynx), crosses over to the heart, then drops down to the stomach.

Damage to the spinal accessory or eleventh cranial nerve will leave you with a shoulder droop. This, because it supplies the long, broad muscle across your back known as the trapezius.

An alcoholic may suffer injury to the hypoglossal nerve. When he opens his mouth, his tongue may seem to be a nest of snakes and wanders all over his mouth. If you injure your twelfth nerve, when you stick out your tongue it will point toward the injured side. This, because the muscle on that part of the tongue has withered and the strong muscle on the uninjured side is pushing the tongue toward the diseased side.

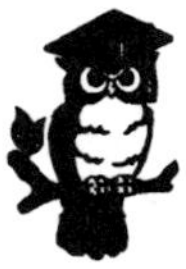

POP QUIZ:9

CRANIAL NERVES

Circle the correct answer

1. The first cranial nerve serves:
   A. taste B. smell C. sight D. hearing

2. The second cranial nerve serves:
   A. taste B. smell C. sight D. hearing

3. The third cranial nerve serves:
   A. taste B. smell C. sight D. eye movement

4. The fourth cranial nerve serves:
   A. taste B. smell C. sight D. eye movement

5. The fifth cranial nerve serves:
A. taste B. sight C. eye movement D. facial sensation

6. The sixth cranial nerve serves:
A. taste B. sight C. eye movement D. facial sensation

7. The seventh cranial nerve serves:
A. taste B. sight C. eye movement D. facial sensation

8. The eighth cranial nerve serves:
A. taste B. sight C. balance D. eye movement

9. The ninth cranial nerves serves:
A. taste B. sight C. balance D. facial movement

10. The tenth cranial nerve serves:
A. ear B. throat C. heart D. all of the above

11. The spinal accessory nerve serves:
A. ear B. throat C. heart D. shoulder

12. The twelfth cranial nerve serves:
A. tongue B. ear C. heart D. lungs

SPINAL CORD

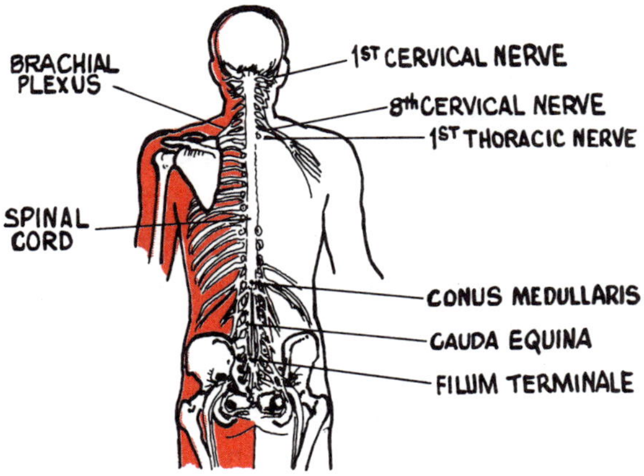

Fig. 43 Spinal Cord

INTRODUCTION

The central nervous system has two main parts: the brain and the spinal cord. We have studied the brain, now we will study the spinal cord.

The spinal cord is about eighteen inches long. It is found in the opening at the center of the back bones. This opening is the **vertebral column**.

The vertebral column continues to grow after the spinal cord has reached its full length. Therefore, the spinal cord does not fill the entire length of the vertebral column.

The vertebral column is about one third longer than the spinal cord.

The spinal cord extends from just above the first neck bone (cervical vertebra), the atlas, at the base of the skull to the level of the first lumbar vertebra. The ending of the spinal cord at the first lumbar vertebra is the **conus medullaris**, or "middle cone." The lumbar vertebra are those in the small of the back. If you bend forward, you may raise the spinal cord even a little more.

In the lower part of the vertebral column, from the end of the spinal cord (conus medullaris), extend long nerve roots. These nerves come from the lower third of the spinal cord. Because of how they look, this group of nerves is called the **cauda equina** ("horse's tail").

Small groups of nerves attached to the spinal cord join to form a series of nerves. Each nerve is made up of a sensory or afferent nerve from the back of the spinal cord and efferent or motor nerve from the front of the spinal cord. In all, there are 31 pairs of spinal nerves.

The nerves leave the vertebral column through spaces between the back bones. They are named for the back bone or vertebra which is just above the space where they exit. As there are 12 thoracic vertebrae, 5 lumbar vertebrae, 5 fused sacral (hip) vertebrae, and 1 to 3 traces of coccygeal (tail) vertebrae, you have 12 thoracic, 5 lumbar, 5 sacral and 1 coccygeal spinal nerves.

You have seven neck bones (cervical vertebrae). But, because one spinal nerve comes out above your first cervical vertebra and one comes out below the last cervical vertebra, you have 8 cervical spinal nerves.

ENLARGEMENTS:

The spinal cord has two enlargements or bulges. There is a cervical enlargement of the spinal cord in the region of the neck. Cervix or cervical means neck. This enlargement is where the fifth through the eighth cervical nerves and the first thoracic nerve emerge. The spinal cord is larger here because these nerves supply the arms and hands. This series of nerves is the "**brachial plexus**." Brachial means arm.

In the lower back is the lumbosacral enlargement. Lumbo means loin or kidney region. These nerves supply the legs and feet.

Meninges: We remember that meninges means membrane. Just as the brain, the spinal cord has three coverings, the meninges. They are, from within outward, the pia mater (tender mother), arachnoid (spider's web) and dura mater (hard mother). These coverings are connected with the same layers surrounding the brain.

The pia mater is closely attached to the spinal cord and holds the blood vessels that supply the cord. After the spinal cord ends, the pia mater continues as a strand in the middle of the cauda equina known as the **filum terminale**. Filum terminale means "end thread." The filum terminale extends to the coccyx.

The second covering is the arachnoid layer. The arachnoid is connected to the pia mater by delicate strands. The region between the pia and the arachnoid is the subarachnoid space. This space is filled with cerebrospinal fluid.

Although the cerebrospinal fluid is formed mostly in the brain, it flows down and around the spinal cord. The fluid cushions the spinal cord.

Below the conus medullaris, the arachnoid forms a blind alley containing the cauda equina and cerebrospinal fluid. It is into this area that needles are inserted to perform a spinal tap. Cerebrospinal fluid is taken out for examination. Also anesthetics may be injected to deaden the lower parts of the body so that surgical operations may be performed without pain. A spinal tap in this area avoids damage to the spinal cord.

The outer meninx is the dura mater. This tough fibrous layer surrounds the cord and then continues over the sheaths of the spinal roots and spinal nerves. It continues below and is attached to the coccyx.

Between the dura mater and the vertebral column is the epidural space. This area contains veins and fat. In the lower sacral region, a hypodermic needle may be inserted into this space for the injection of anesthetics (caudal anesthesia). Caudal anesthesia is used to allow painless child birth.

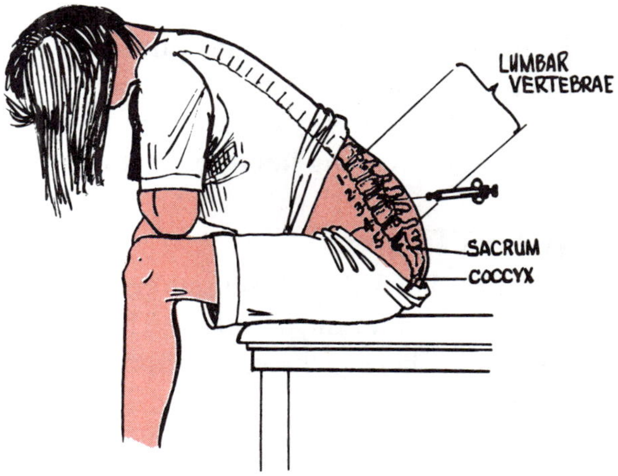

Fig. 44 Spinal Tap

CROSS SECTION:

In cross section the spinal cord looks like an H-shaped or butterfly-shaped center core of gray matter surrounded by white matter. As in the brain, the gray matter is nerve cell bodies with nerve fibers running across it from the white matter and spinal roots.

The white matter is nerve fibers that run up and down the cord. These fibers run up to and down from the brain and other levels of the spinal cord. The whiteness is due to the fatty sheath (myelin sheath) that surrounds many of the fibers. Some glue-like or neuroglia cells which help hold the nerve cells and fibers together are found in both the gray matter and the white matter.

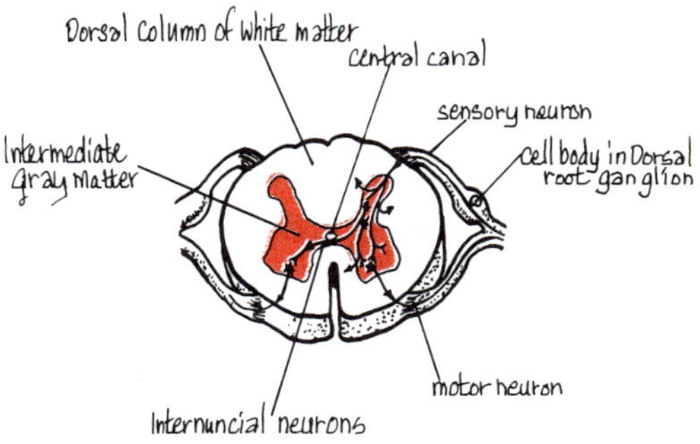

Fig. 45 Cross Section Of Spinal Cord

The arms of the H or wings of the butterfly that stretch toward the back of the body are the **dorsal** or **sensory horns**. The arms of the H or wings of the butterfly that stretch toward the front of the body are the **ventral** or **motor horns**. The crossbar of the H or body of the butterfly is the **gray commissure** or intermediate gray.

There are some neurons in the gray matter whose only job is to send signals from one side of the cord to the other. These are intercalated, internuncial or **interneurons**. The interneurons are the means by which something happening on one side of the body may be felt on the other side of the brain. Also, because of connections provided by the interneurons, something happening to one side of the brain may cause a reaction on the other side of the body.

As the spinal cord itself bulges in the regions of the cervical and lumbosacral enlargements, the gray matter is also largest in these regions because of the large number of nerves necessary to supply the arms, hands, legs and feet.

In the middle of the crossbar or gray commissure is a small opening, the **central canal.** The central canal contains cerebrospinal fluid and communicates with the large ventricles or fluid-filled cavities within the brain.

Surrounding the H-shaped or wings and body of the butterfly appearing gray matter is the white matter. The white matter is subdivided into four columns: the **dorsal column**, between the dorsal horns of the gray matter; the **ventral column**, between the ventral horns of the gray matter; and the **lateral columns**, at the sides of the gray matter.

The white matter has fibers that send nerve impulses from the body (below the head) to the brain and from the brain to the body. The white matter can be divided into zones called **tracts** or pathways. A tract is a collection of nerve fibers having the same origin, job, and ending. Those fibers sending impulses **toward** the brain belong to sensory, or ascending tracts; those sending impulses **from** the brain are motor, or descending, tracts.

SENSATION:

PROPRIOCEPTIVE sensations or feelings are those that give information about movement or position of the body. This information is sent by the fibers in the dorsal white columns. These include: **position sense,** that is, whether you are right side up or up side down and, with your eyes closed, whether your arm is up or down; **pressure sense,** whether you receive a hardy handshake or a wet noodle; **vibratory sense, sense of movement,** and **stereognosis.** When a vibrating tuning fork is placed in the middle of your forehead, you perceive vibratory sense. Stereognosis is two-point discrimination. That is, being able to tell the weight, form, and shape of objects and to tell how far apart two places are when you are touched.

These feelings are sent by fibers that go from the peripheral nerves into the **dorsal** horn of the spinal cord. The main axon of the nerve then goes into the dorsal column on the same side to go up to the lower medulla of the brain.

PAIN and TEMPERATURE feelings go by another pathway. The fibers from the skin, bones, or other organs enter the dorsal horn of the spinal cord. Here, their end branches react with other neurons and send axons **across** the midline to the opposite side to the **lateral white columns**. The fibers then end in the thalamus on the **opposite** side of the brain. Impulses from the thalamus then go to the cerebral cortex.

So what we have is that deep touch and body position are felt on the same side of the brain as they occur in the body. However, feelings of pain and temperature are felt in the opposite side of the brain than where they occur in the body. If you should cut half-way through your spinal cord, then, on the side below the cut, you could not feel deep touch or, with your eyes closed, tell the position of body parts. However, on the side opposite the cut, you could not feel pain or if something was hot or cold. Above the cut everything would still be normal.

MOVEMENT (MOTOR):

MOTOR PATHS

We have studied the gray matter in the dorsal or back part of the spinal cord. These are the dorsal horns. The dorsal horns deal with sensations such as pain and temperature.

The front (ventral) wings or front legs of the butterfly or "H" shaped gray matter in the spinal cord are the **motor horns**. This gray matter is made up of large cells. The axons of these motor neurons pass through the ventral roots to the spinal nerves. They then go to voluntary muscles. They are called lower motor neurons.

Ventral horn motor neuron axons are the only ones that conduct impulses to skeletal muscles. If the lower motor neuron cells are harmed because of injury or disease, they become nonfunctional. In this case, the muscles to which they go receive no stimulation. The muscles then do not contract. The brain cannot make them act nor can they respond to reflexes. They are paralyzed. The muscles shrivel up and waste away. This is called **atrophy**. The series of events is known as lower motor neuron paralysis. Conditions which may cause lower motor neuron paralysis are poliomyelitis (Polio), injury, and tumors.

Neuron cells in the cerebral cortex send axons down the spinal cord to control bodily muscles and organs. Because the cells start in the brain and go down the spinal cord, they are called **corticospinal tracts**.

Axons from the cerebral cortex that come together in the medulla are also called **pyramidal tracts**. They are called pyramidal tracts because they form a bulge or "pyramid" on each side of the front surface (ventral) of the medulla.

After meeting in the medulla, three-fourths of the fibers cross over (decussate) to the other side of the cord and then continue down the cord in the lateral white column. One fourth of the corticospinal fibers do not cross over. Instead, they go down the spinal cord on the same side as that from which they arise. One pair of uncrossed tracts goes down the cord in the lateral white column and one pair goes down in the ventral white column.

When they get to where they are going in the spinal cord, most corticospinal tract fibers do not synapse directly with the anterior horn neurons. Instead they synapse with gray cells called interneurons, which, as we have seen, are cells that lie just within the gray matter and connect two cells.

The job of the pyramidal tracts is to cause individual muscles to move. This is especially important in the hands and the feet. Thus, when your brain wants you to move your big toe, impulses run down the pyramidal tract into the spinal cord and then to the toe muscles.

There are some fibers that come from the brain but do not travel in the pyramidal tracts. These are the extrapyramidal tracts. Some important extrapyramidal tracts come from the reticular formation in the brain stem. These tracts are important in coordinating group muscle movements such as in swimming, running, balance, or smiling.

The brain cells whose axons are in either the pyramidal or extrapyramidal tracts are **upper motor neurons**. Injury to these cells causes spastic paralysis. A spasm is a contraction of a muscle, a "charlie horse." Because many nerve fibers cross, when a person has a clot or hemorrhage of the brain (stroke), muscles on the other side of the body may show spastic paralysis. In this case, the muscles are very rigid and the arm may be moved only with difficulty. If you tapped the patient's knee, his leg might fly straight out. On the other hand, injury to the spinal cord will result in a paralysis on the same side as the injury.

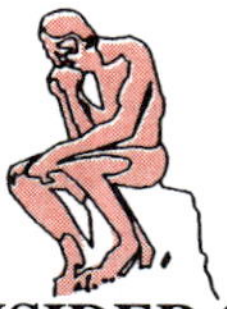

CONSIDER 26:23

HANGMAN'S FRACTURE

Hanging, a common method of execution, began centuries ago and is still performed in some places, although, in this country, hangings are rarely done. Because of automobile accidents, some people suffer injuries that are identical to those observed in hangings. These are called "hangman's fractures." As such, they deserve study.

In hanging, the ideal is sudden death due to disruption of nerves from the brain to the heart and lungs. This is best accomplished by fracture of the base of the brain or the first two neck vertebrae. The place on the victim's head the knot on the noose is positioned is important, as is the weight of the victim and the length of the drop.

During the Roman Empire, executioners simply placed a noose around the victim's neck and hoisted him from the ground. This resulted in a slow death by strangulation and restriction of blood flow to the brain.

In 1784, in an attempt to standardize hanging and prevent slow deaths by strangulation, the "long drop" was adopted. Unfortunately the long drop was not standardized, and when two men were executed with a drop of fifteen feet, one man's head was completely pulled off and the other was partially decapitated.

Because of these problems, more careful attention was taken to study the corpses of people who had been executed by hanging. Study was made as to the weight of the victim and the length of drop necessary to achieve a broken neck.

Of much importance was the placement of the knot. It was discovered that the best place to put the hangman's knot was under the chin. With this placement, the head is hyperextended and the second neck bone (axis) slides forward away from the remainder of the spinal column. Death is instant.

This brings us to the point. Spondylolisthesis of the Axis, or hangman's fracture, which occurs in hanging, is also common in car accidents. The victims head flies forward, strikes the windshield and then is thrown violently backward. Fortunately, if you don't die on the spot, your chances, without surgery, of complete recovery are good.

What do you think of the hangman's fracture? Do you think it poses a good argument for wearing a seat belt with a shoulder harness?

****

SUMMARY
SPINAL CORD

The brain and spinal cord are the two parts of the central nervous system. In an adult, the spinal cord is about eighteen inches long. It fills two-thirds of the vertebral column and extends from the base of the skull to the level of the first lumbar vertebra.

The end of the spinal cord is the conus medullaris or middle cone. The nerves extending from the lower parts of the spinal cord is the horse's tail. There is an enlargement of the spinal cord where nerves for the arm and hands come off and another enlargement for the leg nerves.

As with the brain, the spinal cord is enclosed by the three meninges: pia, arachnoid and dura. Below the conus medullaris, the arachnoid forms a spinal fluid-filled sac from which fluid is obtained by a spinal tap.

On cross section, the gray matter of the spinal cord has the appearance of a butterfly or the letter "H." The back or dorsal gray horns of the spinal cord are where sensory neurons are located. The front or ventral horns of the spinal cord deal with movement and are motor neurons.

Surrounding the gray matter of the spinal cord is the white matter. The white matter is made up of axons either going to or from the brain.

Some sensations, such as pain and temperature, interact with interneurons, called also intercalated or internuncial neurons. These relay neurons allow the sensations to cross to the other side of the spinal cord so that they may be felt on the opposite side of the brain. Three quarters of the axons coursing from the brain down the spinal cord also cross to the other side.

Injury to the brain, such as from a stroke, will commonly cause spastic paralysis to the opposite side of the body. Injury to the spinal cord will most commonly cause a paralysis to the same side of the body below the injury.

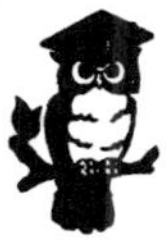

POP QUIZ:10
SPINAL CORD

Circle the correct answer

1. In an adult, the spinal cord is about:
   A. one foot long B. eighteen inches long C. two feet long
   D. eight inches long

2. The end of the spinal cord is the:
   A. conus medullaris B. filum terminale C. cauda equina D. foramina

3. The spinal cord has how many meningeal coverings:
   A. one B. two C. three D. four

4. The spinal cord has how many enlargements:
   A. one B. two C. three D. four

5. The gray matter in the spinal cord is:
   A. "W" shaped B. "Y" shaped C. "H" shaped D. "O" shaped

6. The dorsal horns of the spinal cord deal with:
   A. sensation B. movement C. sight D. hearing

7. The dorsal horns of the spinal cord are:
   A. efferent B. afferent C. motor D. auditory

8. The ventral horns of the spinal cord deal with:
   A. sensation B. movement C. sight D. hearing

9. The ventral horns are:
   A. efferent B. afferent C. sensation D. hearing

10. Fluid for a spinal tap is obtained below the conus medullaris from the:
    A. cauda equina B. filum terminale
    C. subarachnoid space D. central canal

REFLEXES

Sometimes we do things without getting instructions from the brain. These are "reflex" actions. If someone hits you on the knee, your leg may kick out. What has happened is that when your knee was hit, it stretched a tendon. A shock went along the nerves to your spinal cord and then back to the muscles in your leg that causes it to kick.

When your brain catches on to what has happened, it sends a message to your leg to stop kicking. In this case, your brain stops or "inhibits" the action of the spinal cord. If your head were cut off, you would keep kicking.

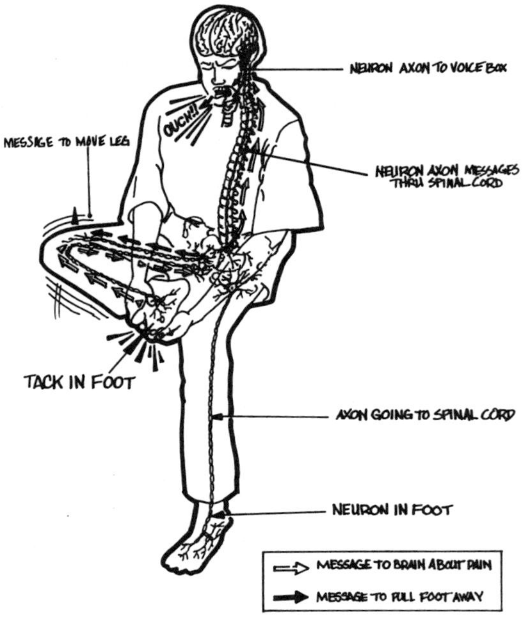

Fig. 46 Reflex Mechanism

CLASS TASK 26:1
KNEE JERK

Take a few minutes. Join into groups of three or four. You are to study the knee jerk reflex.

Have a student sit with his legs crossed. Just below the round area of the knee is a softer area. This is the patellar tendon. Using a ruler or the edge of your hand, strike this tendon a sharp quick blow. You will see the leg fly forward.

It is not necessary to strike very hard. To do so may hurt your friend and show you to be a poor student.

Why did the leg fly forward? What path did the nerve follow to cause this to happen? If the tendon is struck several times, what do you notice? If the subject had no head, what would happen to this reflex? Why?

****

SUMMARY REFLEXES

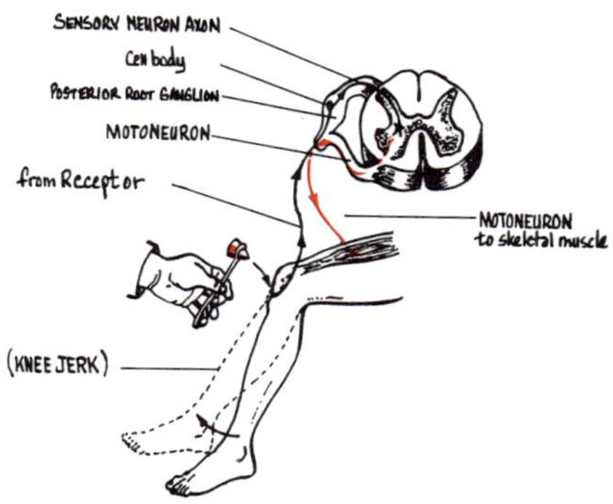

Fig. 47 Knee Jerk Reflex

Reflexes are actions which occur without immediate direction from the brain. If you blink when something comes near your eye, that is a reflex. If you jump when someone says "Boo!" that is a reflex.

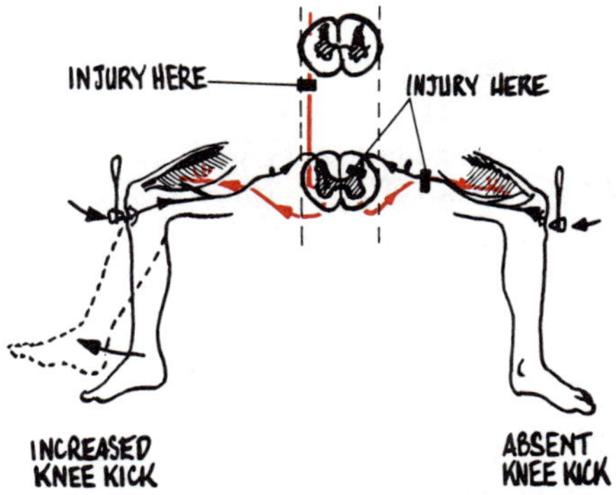

Fig. 48 Reflex Injury

Reflexes may involve only two neurons such as an afferent and an efferent neuron. In more complicated reflexes, more nerves may be involved.

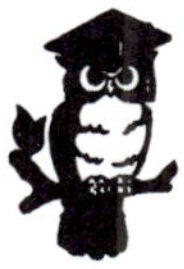

POP QUIZ:11
REFLEXES

True or False

1. Actions occurring without apparent instructions from the brain are called reflexes:
   T F

2. In most reflexes, the brain provides mostly an inhibitory function:
   T F

****

INDEX

A

B

C

D

E